THE 4 SEASON SOLUTION

COAUTHORED BY
DALLAS HARTWIG

The Whole30

It Starts with Food

THE
4 SEASON
SOLUTION

The Groundbreaking New Plan for Feeling Better,
Living Well, and Powering Down Our Always-On Lives

DALLAS HARTWIG

ATRIA BOOKS

New York   London   Toronto   Sydney   New Delhi

ATRIA
BOOKS

An Imprint of Simon & Schuster, Inc.
1230 Avenue of the Americas
New York, NY 10020

First Atria Books hardcover edition March 2020

ATRIA BOOKS and colophon are trademarks of Simon & Schuster, Inc.

For information about special discounts for bulk purchases, please contact Simon & Schuster Special Sales at 1-866-506-1949 or business@simonandschuster.com.

The Simon & Schuster Speakers Bureau can bring authors to your live event. For more information or to book an event, contact the Simon & Schuster Speakers Bureau at 1-866-248-3049 or visit our website at www.simonspeakers.com.

Interior design by Joy O'Meara
Illustrations © Alexis Seabrook

Manufactured in the United States of America

1 3 5 7 9 10 8 6 4 2

Library of Congress Cataloging-in-Publication Data has been applied for.

ISBN 978-1-9821-1515-9
ISBN 978-1-9821-1517-3 (ebook)

CONTENTS

INTRODUCTION

In 1975, a few years before I was born, my parents bought a very small, century-old log cabin in the rural township of Merrickville in eastern Ontario, Canada. It actually wasn't much of a log cabin. The roof had caved in, and a porcupine was living inside. Still, the land was scenic, mostly wooded, with a few fields that had been cleared by hand about one hundred years earlier. My parents politely asked the porcupine to leave, and for that first summer they lived in the old barn until they could make the cabin habitable again. Then they moved in and made it their home.

As pragmatic, countercultural young adults in the early 1970s, their idea was to live simply, away from the rat race of hectic, urban civilization, and that's exactly what they proceeded to do, continuing this lifestyle even after my sister and I came along. When I say that we lived away from civilization, I'm not exaggerating. The cabin was located on one hundred acres at the very end of a dead-end dirt road, many miles from the nearest store or town. Even after it was renovated, it had no electricity or running water. Today, people grumble if they're without the internet for an hour, but we had to pump our water by hand. Showers? Forget about it—we took baths every so often in a tin washtub.

We heated the house with firewood cut from the property, and our single modern luxury was a propane-powered lantern. Oh, and we had an outhouse—not terribly appealing during those frigid Ontario winters. We grew much of our food in a vegetable garden, eating a vegetarian diet and preserving a lot of the food we grew for later months. We had chickens for eggs and goats for milk. A couple of days a week, my mom drove to a town nearby to work at a part-time job. My dad stayed home full time to tend to the house, take care of us kids, keep the garden going, cut wood, and perform other essential tasks. My sister and I spent most of our days outside, exploring the woods, playing with our dog and cat, reading, and daydreaming.

Throughout each day, we lived in sync with the natural rhythms all around us. Because our only light came from oil lamps, the woodstove, and our single, luxurious propane lantern, we organized our schedule according to the sun's movement. When the sun rose, we got up. When it set, we wound down and headed to bed. During the winter, this meant that we slept a great deal, since there wasn't much we could do in the dim light of an oil lamp. In general, our life became much quieter and more intimate during the winter months. In the cold, dark winter we appreciated the warmth of the fire, and the close connections with each other. The summer was totally different: it was light outside until nine or ten o'clock, so we were much more energetic and physically active, and we slept less.

I had no inkling of it as a child, but in living according to nature's rhythms, we were living the way human beings have been doing for most of our history. For most of human history, our ancestors existed as hunters and gatherers, roaming in small bands and living in close contact with their natural surroundings.[1] They were not "living off the land," but rather were *part of* the land. Only about ten thousand to twelve thousand years ago did our Homo sapiens ancestors gradually transition to agricultural societies, with permanent settlements, commerce, and "civilization" arising shortly afterward.[2] The developments in manufacturing and mechanization following the Industrial Revolution (ca. 1740–1840) only took us farther from the earth's natural rhythms. For the last several hundred years, human beings have gravitated to urban centers, as our eating and lifestyle habits have largely been determined by factory timetables and economic efficiency considerations instead of what is optimal for human wellness.[3] Like my own family, a band of ancient hunter-gatherers woke with the rising sun, were active and apart during the day, and reconnected in the evening before going to sleep after it got dark. Over the course of the year, they stayed in tune with seasonal variations. Rather, they *lived* in tune with those variations. There was no other option.

But it wasn't just food and sleep behaviors that followed natural patterns. It was *everything.* In their diet, their physical movements, and their social interactions, too, our ancestors (and modern-day primitive tribes) stayed in tune with the rhythms of nature—eating different foods in different seasons (and in different places), moving their bodies in different ways at different times based on the demands of their environment, and exploring their world freely at times and staying closer to the safety and familiarity of the tribe at other times. The whole arc of their lives followed a pattern that mirrored the seasons of a year: they were born; they budded into adolescence and bloomed into adulthood; they contributed to the tribe through physical labor and sharing wisdom; they shared their lifetime of accumulated wisdom with the rest of the tribe, planting seeds for a better next generation; and eventually they died, often at a very advanced age. Of course, many of our ancestors died prematurely due to infant mortality, accidents, infection, or acts of violence—I'm not trying to paint a romanticized picture. But in general, their lives were rhythmic and circular, even leisurely, not because they wished them so, but because that's the way it was for people so immediately dependent on and immersed in nature. Research shows us that contemporary hunter-gatherers actually have considerably more leisure time than we do in our modern, convenience-laden, productivity-oriented society.[4]

My family, of course, didn't *have* to live so close to nature. And in 1983, when I turned five, we pretty much stopped doing it. We closed up our cabin, sold our land, and moved closer to a small town called Brockville. Although we still lived in a rural setting (on an apple orchard outside of town), we adopted a more conventional way of life. Our new house had electricity and running water, and I attended a small school with other kids from town. By and large, I left behind my intimate connection with nature and those seasonal rhythms. I finished elementary and high school, attended university in the United States, earned a degree in anatomy and physiology and a graduate degree in physical therapy, and lived in a number of places in the country. I was always attentive to healthy living—I ate well (conventionally speaking), played competitive volleyball, climbed mountains, and rode mountain bikes. But I didn't think much about natural living per se, and my own personal habits were as artificial and disconnected from natural rhythms as most people's.

That began to change in 2007, when my father passed away prematurely of pancreatic cancer. Deeply impacted by his death, I began to look at my life in new ways, and to question many of my lifestyle choices. I was a healthy twentysomething, working in a profession that

I enjoyed. I was lean and fit, eating in ways that most people would consider healthy, and blessed with a strong network of friends. Anybody who met me would have considered me the very picture of health. But the reality was more complicated. Deep down, I sensed that not all was right. I was working too hard and obviously not getting enough sleep. I had some adult acne, and chronic inflammation in my left shoulder. I felt stressed and overstimulated, and while I thought I was more or less "happy," I also felt adrift, lacking a deeper sense of peace and rootedness. I had lots of friends, but still felt pretty isolated. What was I really doing with my life?

Always intellectually curious, I read a number of books and research papers that cued me in to our evolutionary past and its enormous relevance for our present-day health. I became especially fascinated with the idea of physiological rhythms and began chasing down anything I could find in the scientific literature on that topic. There was quite a lot of research out there—hundreds of published papers that I eventually read and analyzed. What I discovered fascinated me.

Biologically, we're walking around in bodies that are well adapted to gathering seasonal plants and hunting ancient animals, sleeping deeply during the hours of darkness, and living and working together as a tight-knit tribe—bodies, in other words, that operate on nature's clock and *expect* cyclical variations in our key lifestyle behaviors. All of our physiological systems and even individual cells have internal mechanisms that align us with nature's oscillations between on and off, active and resting, open and closed, expansion and contraction. More tangibly, rhythmic patterns are encoded on the molecular level in the DNA of (almost) all living things, even single-cell organisms that lack a nervous system and the ability to communicate in complex ways.[5] Rhythms are perceptible everywhere. We are not on/off creatures. We fluctuate and flow. We expand and contract.

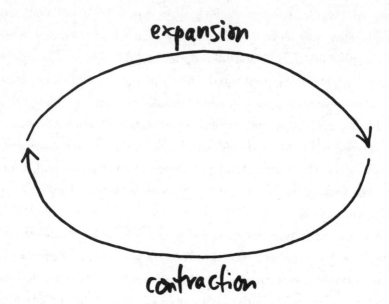

expansion

contraction

As I came to realize, our bodies are at odds with everyday conditions and schedules in the modern world, which tend to be linear and binary rather than cyclical and gradual. Today, alarm clocks and artificial lights give us control over how we structure our days, so we can stay up far into the night and wake up long before (or long after) sunrise. Modern agriculture and global commerce allow us to eat whatever we want, no matter the time of year. Whereas our ancestors had to walk, run, climb, and carry things during the daylight hours in order to survive, we can live sedentary lives and still put food on the table and a roof over our heads. Nor are we dependent, as our ancestors were, on a close-knit tribe in order to thrive. Many of us live atomized lives, separated from our families and friends by large distances. Our days rarely echo the ancient patterns of social interaction—broad contact with others during the daytime, retreating into a smaller, more intimate circle at night. Instead, some of us feel socially isolated for much of the day *and* night. We keep ourselves so busy during our waking hours and distracted just before and after sleep that we don't allow ourselves the kinds of opportunities our ancestors did to reconnect with the person who matters most—ourselves. The nonstop external stimulation displaces the quietude and openness necessary for us to know and deeply care for our own inner worlds.

The science I was reading during those early years suggested that modernity's deviation from natural rhythms had exacted a huge, and largely unremarked upon, toll on human health. Since we don't eat seasonally and locally, and we rely on shelf-stable processed foods, we don't get the nutrition we need—a variable mix of protein, fat, carbohydrates, and micronutrients. We often wind up eating too little complete protein and too much refined carbohydrate and sugar. Over time, this unbalanced, nutrient-poor diet causes our stress-induced cravings for sugar and carbohydrates to intensify. We never feel that we have eaten enough, and no matter how much we eat, we still want more. We wind up sick with chronic illnesses like cancer, heart disease, and obesity.

The shift from traditional, whole-food diets to modern, processed foods is a central cause of these "diseases of civilization." But it's not the only cause. We also don't get the sleep we need throughout the year, leaving ourselves vulnerable to addiction to caffeine or alcohol, which we consume in order to compensate—to wake us up or calm us down. Inadequate sleep also leaves us more vulnerable to insomnia, mental illness like anxiety and depression, heart disease, cancer, and other chronic diseases. And it's not just the sleep itself. As I explain in the following pages, it's also the amount of time we spend in darkness or near-darkness that directly impacts our health.

We also don't move our bodies in tune with the rhythms of nature as they're evolved to do, so we either stay sedentary and develop related chronic diseases, or we cajole ourselves into exercising in highly contrived ways, leaving us vulnerable to injuries or other stress-related problems. While the modern features of low-nutrient processed food, sedentary and overstimulating lifestyles, and chronically disrupted circadian rhythms are most certainly problematic, there is yet another direct influence on our overall health and quality of life that is emerging as massively impactful: loneliness and social isolation. We feel disconnected from others, so we turn to social media as a panacea for loneliness and as a facsimile for deep companionship—which makes us feel even more disconnected. We fall prey to depression, anxiety, substance abuse, and worse. We lose touch with our four primary lifestyle variables—sleep, eat, move, and connect—that are essential to living well. In contrast to our hunter-gatherer ancestors, who slept, ate, moved, and connected according to annual seasonal changes, today we sleep poorly and erratically, move infrequently or excessively, eat processed, nutrient-poor, and inflammatory foods, and connect artificially while remaining essentially isolated. This creates a closed loop, a self-perpetuating cycle, because the less we exercise or the more stress we experience or the more poorly we sleep, the more we turn to "comforting" processed foods and stimulating media that in turn further disrupt our sleep or contribute to inflammatory health issues, priming us to scroll through social media late at night (instead of connecting vulnerably with an actual person), leaving us feeling less-than, left out, and often very, very alone. The brilliant Austrian psychologist Viktor Frankl is often credited with saying, "When a person can't find a deep sense of meaning, they distract themselves with pleasure."[6] Is this not the everyday experience for many of us? Individually and collectively, we have not made seeking our life's meaning a priority (in part because we've been conditioned by cultural norms), thus opening ourselves up to pleasure seeking and addictions of all flavors as ways of coping with feeling adrift and without direction. Additionally, our civilization is built on pervasive themes of expansion, consumption, stimulation, self-gratification, and the "pursuit of happiness," which only serves to alienate us from that deeper sense of meaning and contribution that could act as our North Star, our guiding light.

While we may be living *longer* than our prehistoric ances- tors, we are not living *better*; research suggests that we are getting sicker and living less satisfying lives. In fact, the more I read about our modern disconnection from natural rhythms, the more I found myself increasingly questioning, as Thomas Paine did back in 1795, "whether . . . civilization has most promoted or most injured the general happiness of man . . ."[7]

Despite our growing recognition of the problems with modernity, the solution isn't to turn back the clock of human history, giving up our houses, electricity, cars, and smartphones, and instead choosing a primitive hunter-gatherer way of life. Why would we want to do that? Even if it were possible, which it isn't, we would be foolish to part with some of the powerful and enriching technology humanity has developed through the agricultural, industrial, and digital revolutions. But then again, back in 2006, it also would have been foolish of me to carry on with my "modern" approach to "healthy" living. As it turns out, I didn't.

An Experiment in Living Better

Many years ago, I wondered if perhaps my sense of malaise and dis- connection would improve if I started to pay more attention to my body's intrinsic rhythms. In falling into my early adult lifestyle, I had largely accepted at face value what modern society told me to do to stay healthy and happy, but it wasn't working. Maybe I could live better by breaking with convention and taking some small steps, guided by research and my own intuition, to become more in tune with my body's oscillating needs.

My first move was to experiment with changing how I ate. Influenced in particular by writers like Michael Pollan, I broke from our industrialized food system and began trying to eat locally, which by definition meant eating seasonally.[8] I gave up eating grapes (imported from Chile) in the wintertime, and instead ate lots of leafy greens in the spring, and more hearty stews and root vegetables in the fall. More generally, eating seasonally meant that like our ancestors in temperate climates, I began eating fresher, nutrient-dense, antioxidant-rich plant foods in the spring and summer, when they were readily available, more starchy vegetables and roots in the fall, and heartier protein- and fat-rich foods during the cooler fall and long winter.

I noticed something: the more I chose to eat whole, seasonal foods, the better I felt—not just physically, but emotionally and even spiritually. That in turn sparked me to wonder what more I might accomplish if I adjusted other behaviors so that they were in tune with nature's fluctuations. Beginning around 2008, I went beyond food and came to think about an entire *system* of rhythmic living. I drew on the psychologist Abraham Maslow's theory of the hierarchy of needs. Under his schema, our most basic needs were physiological in nature—the needs for food, water, sleep, and so on. Having met those requirements, people could then go on to satisfy their needs for a sense of security and for strong, intimate, nourishing relationships. Maslow conceived of higher-level needs as well, such as the need for feeling a sense of accomplishment or for feeling spiritually "actualized" as a person—but as he argued, you needed to satisfy lower-order needs before you began ascending the hierarchy.[9]

In conceiving a model for rhythmic living, I focused on those lower-order needs and eventually thought about and researched rhythmic patterns in four distinct areas of life: how we eat, sleep, move (exercise), and connect. I construed the last of these quite broadly, focusing not merely on how we related with others, but also how we related with ourselves and how we felt a sense of connection to a place. Going beyond the more tangible connections to self, place, and others, I also addressed the importance of a deeper sense of purpose—a sense of living well while contributing to something larger than oneself. My working theory was that if I could tune in better to my body's natural rhythms in these areas, then I could improve my overall level of health, eventually freeing myself to satisfy higher-level intellectual, emotional, and spiritual needs.

By about 2010, I had embarked on a broad and flexible experiment to rediscover and reconnect with my own body's natural rhythms. This wasn't a formal, rigidly structured thirty-day kind of plan, but a more fluid, ongoing set of experiments I undertook in concert with my evolving awareness of my body. In addition to continuing to eat locally, I followed my intuition and began to adjust my bedtimes and waking times so that they corresponded to seasonal patterns in the length of the day. This change alone tended to make my physical movements more rhythmic as well as more intuitively satisfying—I now moved most during the late morning and early afternoon, and significantly reduced my intense activity in the evening as the sun was beginning to set. I made my choices of activity more seasonal—weight lifting and interval training in the winter, mountain biking and hiking in the summer. When it came to structured exercise, I went for endurance training (and a lot more general activity, not just formal "exercise") in the summer and shorter, more intense interval training and strength training in the winter to mirror the patterns that, according to my research, our ancestors (at least those in temperate climates) had likely followed.

Introduction

Not surprisingly, the pattern of "building" in the off-season (winter) and "conditioning" in the preseason (spring and summer) is common in competitive summer sports. In those early years of personalizing what I'd learned through my research, I also modified how I engaged with other people at different times of the year, getting out and "expanding my horizons" during the summer months, and "hunkering down" during the winter months and focusing on fewer but far more intimate relationships.

In every way I could think of, I started to honor the natural rhythms, both on the daily and seasonal levels. The deeper I got into it, the more I realized that I had embarked on a journey with some profoundly countercultural implications. Many of us today have a hard time slowing down. We stay in a frenetic, stimulating, always-on, multitasking kind of mode in terms of how we sleep, eat, move, and connect (or . . . don't). Because we're stuck in this pattern of perpetual "summer" behavior, our deepest needs aren't being met, and we feel unsettled and unmoored, adrift in the world of working, trying to have fun, and seeking "happiness." We often become addicted to artificial substitutes for those needs—refined sugar instead of complete protein, caffeine instead of restful sleep, daily spin classes instead of picking up heavy things, social media instead of real, face-to-face contact. In the broadest sense, we're even addicted to this kind of fast-paced existence itself, maintaining it even though we notice that it exhausts us, leaves us out of balance, and ultimately threatens our health. It feels good and bad at the same time, but we simply don't know what to do differently. This is just what we're supposed to do, right?

In my experiments, I sped my life up at certain times but slowed down at others, as our ancestors did. I made my life more intense and challenging at certain points, and much more restorative and restful at others. I aimed for excitement and adventure and growth at certain times, calmness and placidity and quiet withdrawal at others. I was still living what most people would consider a "normal" life, but beneath the surface I was doing many things very differently than others around me. The more I experimented, the more I saw the ancient wisdom of a more natural, oscillatory way of life. And the more I learned about natural rhythms, the more I experimented. A positive dynamic took hold that left me feeling more energetic and creative, but also more peaceful, rested, grounded, and connected with others. My mood improved, as did my focus. *Everything* felt better. And I wasn't trying nearly as hard to maintain healthy habits as I had been before. Because I was making incremental changes that felt intuitively right to me and that helped me feel better, I *owned* those changes in a whole new way. How could I *not* behave in these ways, now that I knew that it made me feel deeply better? Living well became far easier and more fun than it had ever been before.

I knew I was onto something, and I was excited to tell others about it. So, I began to present my ideas at academic conferences. My friend and colleague Jamie Scott, a health researcher based in New Zealand, and I presented a talk on the seasonal model for health at the Ancestral Health Symposium to a packed house. The simple-but-profound approach resonated deeply with people, and they told me that I was presenting a new paradigm for thinking about living in a more integrated fashion. They were excited and urged me to write a book on the subject. The momentum was building. And then . . . I did nothing.

Well, not exactly. For a number of years, I put my new, integrative model aside and focused on one particular piece of it, the part dealing with food. Many readers will know me for having coauthored the bestselling books *It Starts with Food* and *The Whole30*. These books, which empowered people to bring their diets in tune with their bodies' innate needs, were key components of my four-part rhythmic model. In 2011, when I was working on *It Starts with Food,* I didn't merely think of the word "it" as meaning "good health." To me, "it" also meant dedication to rhythmically attuned living. If you want to bring your body in harmony with its natural rhythms, you can't do it with the wave of a magic wand, or simply by adhering to a new shopping list. It has to happen incrementally as you learn, unlearn, relearn, and eventually integrate lessons along the way. If you could only pick one place to start, my training, research, and personal experience all told me that this should be diet. It starts—but certainly doesn't end—with food.

The thirty-day Whole30 experiment clearly emphasizes diet. Over a monthlong period, we ask participants to radically change their dietary habits, avoiding all alcohol, legumes, grains, sugars and refined sweeteners, dairy products, and artificial additives (like carrageenan and MSG). In their place, we tell people to stock up on healthy fats, meat, seafood, poultry, veggies of all types, fruit, and nuts and seeds. I always considered this diet part of a larger, fully integrated program of behavior change and self-awareness, aimed at empowering people by helping them rediscover what their own bodies were telling them. That's why we discouraged any "fake treats," like Paleo waffles made from mashed bananas, or pizza crust fashioned from a crushed cauliflower. Consuming such foods followed the letter of the law but definitely not the spirit of the program, which wasn't to imitate conventional or junk food products, but to entirely reimagine your attitude toward food and your own health. It's also why we eliminated all the most commonly problematic foods that cause digestive issues, like gluten and dairy, allowing people to create a clean digestive slate, and then progressively, little by little, to reintroduce certain foods after the thirty days and see how they felt, both physically and emotionally. To be sure, some people who embraced the Whole30 did so because they wanted to attain specific health objectives such as losing weight or relieving disease symptoms, but that was never my deepest intention. With the Whole30 program, I sought to give people some initial tools for becoming more aware of their own bodies' inherent needs, so that they could feel empowered to take steps on their own to satisfy those needs, become healthier, and even more important, live a life of purpose and deep joy. The Whole30 was just the beginning of the beginning.

The 4 Season Solution is the book I imagined writing almost a decade ago—the prequel to *It Starts with Food*, really. The book presents my four-part theory and introduces a groundbreaking health approach that you can deploy immediately to achieve steady, sustainable gains over time. Within my framework, you attend to your health and well-being in a personalized way, on your own terms, and without requiring doctors, coaches, or other outside experts. Whether you've struggled to stay well or you simply want to be living better than you currently are, *The 4 Season Solution* will cast new light on your current health behaviors and how they might be undermining your goals and values. The book will also show you how to start changing those behaviors so that you can progress toward many important goals at once—better sleep, a healthier weight, more energy, brighter skin, deeper meaning and purpose, lower stress, and a greater sense of connectedness, contentment, and peace.

Leaning into Wellness

Many people who completed the Whole30 program have written to me to describe the transformative changes they have seen in their lives—changes that went far beyond the food they eat. For some, the opportunity to learn how their diet affected them individually led them to rethink unhealthy relationships and to improve them. Others were moved to start exercising, stop smoking, go to graduate school, or pursue creative endeavors that they had long neglected. What I've found absolutely fascinating and inspiring is that Whole30 participants consistently took on these higher-order growth opportunities once the roadblock of their unhealthy diet was removed. Repeatedly, people posed this question: "I've changed my diet, and I feel so much better. What can I do next?" Clearing the fog caused by problematic foods allowed them to spontaneously and energetically pursue other avenues of growth and meaningful experiences.

As I knew firsthand, there isn't just one particular change or even a series of discrete changes you can make to achieve optimum health. Living better is an ongoing and never-ending process of behavior change, all grounded in your ability to cue into your body and its rhythmic needs. What was needed, I thought, was a book that presented the larger framework for rhythmically based living, so that others could do what I did: move *yourself* toward better health by changing your behaviors in a way and at a pace that feels right for you.

Unlike *The Whole30*, which offers a highly structured, tightly constrained program for people to follow, *The 4 Season Solution* presents a conceptual road map to explore your own body and health . . . and life! It helps you rethink your health habits from an ancestral and biological standpoint so that you can then reshape them. Who knows where you'll start—or where you'll go—as you learn how our bodies have evolved to function, how we're failing to effectively meet our body's most basic needs, and how our health gets compromised as a result. One thing I do know: the more you learn, and the more you experiment, the more you'll want to learn and experiment. That's because this book prompts you to consult the greatest health expert of all, and one who is most routinely neglected—you. I know a lot about how human bodies work, but I don't know what's best for *your* body. That's for *you* to discover and for you to champion.

Although we might have fallen out of touch with our natural rhythms, all of us intuitively *know* what our bodies need. We have just become habituated to ignore the urges inside us that would cue us to sleep, eat, move, and connect in certain ways at certain times of the day or year. With our intuition consistently ignored and underdeveloped, we rely almost exclusively on our rational selves—and our willpower—to adopt and stick with healthy behaviors. But willpower alone doesn't usually help us stick with health regimens. We all have a limited supply of willpower, and all too frequently, the tank runs empty because we are using it to deal with annoying coworkers, traffic, tempting treats, and strained relationships with friends or partners. Plus, mustering up willpower all the time is *hard*. Your intuition is the path to a healthier, saner, happier, calmer, and more fulfilling life, all with progressively *less* brute effort on your part.

This is not to say that syncing your body with natural rhythms will always be easy. It won't. If you travel every week for your job, sitting for many hours on planes or in cars, you might have some ability to pay more respect to your bodily rhythms, but ultimately, achieving better health might require that you change your life so that you travel less. If you eat pizza multiple times a week because it's cheap and convenient, you might have to spend more on food to improve your diet. You don't have to be independently wealthy to live a healthy life, but you do have to recalibrate how you live, as well as allocate your time and money in ways that echo your personal values in order to respect your body's evolutionary needs. This might mean cutting back on impulsive shopping or getting a cheaper cable TV plan so that you can afford higher-quality, locally produced, organic food. Or it might mean asking your boss to adjust your work schedule seasonally so that you can more closely follow your body's natural sleep rhythms. The point is to become more aware of your rhythms, so that you can understand the impact of your daily behaviors and make conscious decisions about how you live and the level of health you enjoy. Small, sustainable changes in your behavior lead you to better health over months, years, and ultimately, a lifetime. The key is simply to get started somewhere with an experiment of your choosing.

I've organized this book to make it as easy as possible to understand our premodern bodies and to try on new behaviors. The first chapter builds on the behavioral theory of health I've sketched out, detailing several key concepts that will help us understand our collective and problematic disconnection from our bodies. The following four chapters present my model, arguing that for optimal human health the four basic needs—sleep, food, movement, meaningful connection— must align with one another, and that they must oscillate. I've used the phrase "coordinate then oscillate" to succinctly express how to bring these four areas of health behaviors back into harmony with each other. Match, then move. Each of these chapters draws on the latest science to examine our bodies' natural patterns in one of these areas. Comparing these patterns with the demands of modern life, I identify areas of mismatch and explain how they lead to dysfunction, disease, and a general feeling of being "stuck." Chapters 6, 7, and 8 explore how our natural rhythms in the four areas interact during the course of three time periods, respectively: the day, the year, and your entire lifetime. Here I'll help you assess where your daily habits might be going astray from your body's needs, and I'll suggest some behavior change experiments to try. I'll close the book by evoking the "endgame" that long-term dedication can yield: a life of deeper peace, enrichment, and fulfillment beyond the usual bodily cravings that occupy us.

My own health has improved dramatically since I started realigning my behaviors and habits with my internal rhythms. After a decade of experimenting, I understand that my previous ways of sleeping, eating, moving, and connecting left a lot to be desired. At certain times of the year, I now spend less time exercising and more time sleeping. At all times, I eat food seasonally that helps support my exercise program. I've become adept at slowing down and turning inward at certain times, and accelerating and expanding outward at others. Best of all, I've learned to apply rhythmic principles to my social relationships. That means, for example, that I don't throw myself headlong into "holiday party season," since the intense stimulation of parties with co-workers or friends is at odds with our natural autumnal desire to hunker down for the coming winter, to withdraw, to rest. When healing after a painful divorce, I took solace in an extended, symbolic winter season, using it to introspect, develop my self-awareness, and restore my sapped energy.

I've also put sensible limits on my social media use and our always-on culture. While I maintain a large and growing social media following, and enjoy interacting with followers all over the world, I now spend more time connecting deeply with just a few close friends and family members, as well as with myself. My social way of being varies seasonally as well, with more boisterous social engagements in the summertime, and far fewer in the winter. My life is far more satisfying and, in all senses of the word, healthier.

Just as Abraham Maslow's hierarchy of needs would imply, healthier tends to beget happier. Meeting foundational needs such as enough nourishing food and proper synchronization with intrinsic circadian rhythms allows humans to spontaneously and meaningfully address other, higher-order needs, such as those of cognitive and emotional growth, appreciation of beauty and wonderment, and inspiration to impart a legacy to future generations. That is, a sense of contribution and meaning outside one's self. When I do choose to behave in ways that run contrary to my intuitive rhythms, which isn't often, I make that choice consciously and purposefully, aware of both the potential benefits and known costs.

We don't have to part with the comforts of civilization to realize the full, rich, beautiful potential of our existence. Although civilization remains starkly at odds with what we might regard as a "natural state," most of us enjoy more latitude than we might think in acknowledging natural patterns and living in concert with them. Imagine what you might achieve if you broke free of modern life in your thinking, reexamined all of your behaviors and habits looking for those biological mismatches, and began the gradual process of tuning in to your body's innate inclinations. Imagine how you'd grow as you came to cut through all the noise and understand what your body *really* wants at specific times throughout your day and year (and life). Imagine not having to run interference on your cravings and intuitions, understanding and honoring them instead of suppressing and ignoring them, or helplessly caving to them. Imagine how fulfilling it would be to experiment with small behavior tweaks—and to see sustained, quantitative results. It's an incredible adventure, and it's yours for the taking. The solution is upon you.

PART ONE

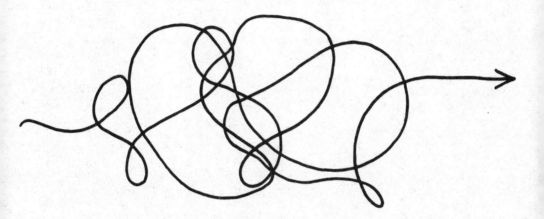

GETTING
STUCK

CHAPTER ONE

Beaten Down by Being Normal

Kim, a woman in her midthirties, consulted with me to discuss her health and how she might improve it. Like so many mothers, her daily schedule was hectic, as she juggled part-time work with family and household demands. Prioritizing helping her children and husband in the morning, she gave little thought to her own breakfast and lunch, and then battled to fit what was effectively a full-time job into her part-time day. Even as we sat down to focus on Kim's own needs, her phone beeped and buzzed with seemingly endless messages from work, her husband, and reminders about events for the kids.

Kim's evenings mirrored her mornings. Dinner needed to be cooked, and the kids wrangled for homework, dinner, and, eventually, bed. If she did manage to get the kids settled and asleep at a reasonable time, she usually spent the remainder of her nights on the couch, engaged in a vague and shifting combination of television watching, messaging friends on her phone, scrolling through Facebook, answering work-related emails, or "window shopping" for items she didn't really need. Her husband sometimes sat with her, engaged in similar activities of his own, but more often lingered on his computer elsewhere in the house catching up on his own work.

Kim thought of the relationships in her life as "good," but not great. She and her husband both felt committed to their marriage and tried to schedule some sort of a "date night" once a week, although the kids and their general lack of energy and enthusiasm often undermined that plan. Struggling to meet everyday demands, Kim and her husband didn't connect deeply with each other much. Their sex life was mediocre, mostly because neither of them felt particularly energetic in the evening once the kids had finally settled into bed, and because they were essentially in survival mode much of the time.

Their relationship with the kids, like their relationship with each other, was not terrible, but not great, either. They faithfully attended parent-teacher conferences and looked after their kids' academic needs and social lives, but they weren't truly connecting. Case in point: Kim and her husband made it a priority to eat dinner most nights together as a family, but found it was such a battle to get the kids off their electronic devices that they eventually abandoned their *no devices at dinner* policy altogether. It just wasn't worth the arguments and stress it caused everyone.

Physically, Kim wasn't in terrible shape, but she'd lost the healthy, glowing "athlete's body" she had maintained earlier in life. As she told me, she suffered from "the usual" back and knee aches, tension headaches, and her main concern, crashing energy levels. She felt physically and emotionally "fragile," she said, and believed the answer (and her reason for seeking my advice) was to go to the gym three times per week and start exercising. She imagined doing some cardio on the bike and treadmill. When I inquired as to when she might fit this in, she said she thought she could do it over the winter months, after 8:30 p.m., once the kids were settled in bed. Kim was looking for help, but her perceptions about where to begin shifting were mismatched to what was actually causing her deteriorating physical and mental health. She was confused and discouraged but still trying to make things better, hence her consultation with me.

Does Kim's story sound familiar? It should. Although "Kim" isn't a real person, her story echoes hundreds of others I've heard throughout my years of coaching. Like her, most of us feel less healthy than we'd like—tired, overwhelmed, distracted, "fragile," mired in uninspiring relationships. We want to fix things, so we try diets and exercise regimens and meditation, but nothing seems to work—or at least, not for very long, and not in the comprehensive way that we were hoping for.

Kim's is the all-too-common story of the daily grind of modern life—where every day of the year, for years on end, is virtually the same. Modern life, in modern consumer cultures at least, has flattened out, averaged, or disregarded many of the oscillations, rhythms, and cycles of the natural world (and our evolutionary past). Sunrise might vary by three or more hours between summer and winter solstices, but your alarm still goes off at 5:15 every morning *as regularly as clockwork*. Seasonal temperature variations have been replaced with climate control systems in our homes, cars, and workplaces. No matter where you are, or what season you are in, it is always 65 to 72°F (18 to 22°C). If you fancy mangoes in the midst of winter, no problem. Pre-ripened picking, packing, and global shipping can bring you any tropical fruit your sweet tastes desire, even when it is literally freezing outside. And you can go to your gym and run on the treadmill under fluorescent lights at nearly any time of the day or night.

It feels great to have the food we like continuously available and to not experience temperature extremes, but this modern "flattening" also has a serious downside. As with Kim, it's left us "stuck" in a mix of incongruent health behavior, like maintaining hectic summer-style schedules in the depths of winter. The good news is, our natural rhythms haven't been lost. They're still there, temporarily buried but surprisingly accessible, waiting to be rediscovered and to direct you toward a more natural and effortless way of being in the world.

Our Bodies, Our Rhythms

Let's say I plucked you and a group of your closest friends and loved ones out of our standardized, modern existence and dropped you all on a Jurassic Park–style island (we'll say sans dinosaurs for now). You have no access to any of life's modern conveniences, and in particular, no access to clocks, watches, calendars, or any other modern way of marking time. How would you keep track of the passing days?

Chances are, within a very short period of time—quite literally, hours—you would hook back into one of life's many natural rhythms. In the absence of bright lights, Netflix, smartphones, and so on, you and your island clan would likely head to bed not long after sundown, with nothing to wind you up except for the occasional brightness of a full moon. You would quickly learn to mark the progression of the days via the sun's rising and setting. You might track the progression of the year by following the sun's arc in the sky—low in winter, high in summer. In this way, you would soon be able to mark the solstices— the point at which the sun changes its trajectory and the days become shorter or longer, cooler or warmer. Approximately halfway between the solstices, you'd have an equinox, where day and night are roughly equal in length. You would also track the months and progression of the year via the repeating phases of the moon—the lunar cycles. You might notice changes in plant life, flowers and fruit, weather patterns, and animal behaviors as indications of changes in the seasons. The longer you remained isolated from modernity, the more likely you would be in tune with, and live by, such rhythms.

Within yourself, in the absence of caffeine, sugar, alcohol, artificial light, and all the other common stimulants we use to *get through life*, you might begin to notice a certain rhythmicity to your own energy levels. You might become spontaneously active and exploratory in the early part of the day but seek a comfortable spot to take a siesta in the early afternoon. You might perk up again in the late afternoon and into the early evening but find yourself wanting to head to sleep not that long after sundown, and certainly much earlier than you would in your modern, electronic home. Spring and summer might find you and your tribe using the longer day length and warmth to explore your surroundings further, attempting to learn what was over that mountain, or beyond the horizon. Autumn and winter might see you lingering a little closer to your base camp, hunkering down on the shorter, cooler days, and making the most of the bounty of resources you had stockpiled during the warmer months. Winter would mean less exploration and activity, and more recovery and planning ahead.

Year upon year, you'd see these rhythms organically ebb and flow, expand and contract. If you experienced your particular environment long enough, you might begin to notice rhythms in longer time frames, such as climate rhythms—how every five years or so, for example, it might become particularly wet or dry. Some plant or animal might become abundant or scarce on a rhythmic basis. Perhaps within your own lifetime, or across the generations, you would accumulate a store of such environmental knowledge and wisdom, and be capable of predicting the frequency of volcanic eruptions, earthquakes, and other natural occurrences. These are just a few examples of some of the many rhythms, short and long, that exist in the natural world and that our ancestors (and thus our own genetic, social, and cultural heritage) would have had exposure to for countless generations. This accumulated wisdom depends on intergenerational respect and the recognition of the value of elders as guardians of invaluable information that cannot be neatly packaged into Wikipedia articles or tweets.

But of course, we don't live in Jurassic Park—and we don't need to in order to sense our natural patterns. Even in the pressure cooker of modern life, they peek through from time to time. When we get restful sleep at night, wake up energized, get into a groove sometime midmorning, and tap into our best productivity, we notice it. We might also notice energy fluctuations throughout the year. Some months we might have boundless energy, while in others we might feel quieter and more contemplative.

Taking such observations seriously and studying our bodily patterns, we find that we aren't just peripherally bound to the ebb and flow of the natural world. Rather, those oscillations are inscribed into our very physiology. We can think of a biological rhythm as any cyclical change in the body's chemistry and/or function. That broad definition includes everything from our daily sleep cycles, to the regulation of our body temperature, to the menstrual cycle. To use the technical lingo, these rhythms are *endogenous*—controlled by an internal and self-sustaining biological clock.

Body temperature is a good example. You might remember from high school health class that our "natural" temperature is 98.6°F. But that's just a baseline, as our body temperature fluctuates throughout the day. During our waking hours, it gradually rises several degrees, hitting its highest point around 4:00 to 6:00 p.m. The body's lowest temperature comes in the early morning, hours before we wake up.[1] That's useful to know, as we feel our most energetic as our body temperature increases throughout the day, and we feel more relaxed and sleepy as our temperature falls in the evening and nighttime.[2]

Decreasing temperatures signal to your body that it's time to slow down and prepare for sleep. We sleep in cycles, too, all of which are roughly ninety minutes long. When we enter our most intensive, rapid-eye-movement (REM) periods of our sleep, the cells controlling our temperature temporarily deactivate.[3] That means our surroundings determine our body temperature during REM. If you're missing some needed shut-eye, or if you wake up frequently at night, it might be that your bedroom is too warm.[4] Consider lowering the thermostat a few degrees. Or, better yet, ditch those pajamas and sleep *au natural*. Unfortunately, modern environmental exposures, as well as stress and anxiety, can influence and disrupt these endogenous rhythms as well.

In addition to internal, self-activating cues, our bodies also have external or *exogenous* rhythms, biological cycles that harmonize with external stimuli. Such external stimuli are referred to as *zeitgebers*, from the German word meaning "time givers." Zeitgebers help to keep the biological clock synchronized to a twenty-four-hour period and include environmental time prompts such as sunlight, food, noise, and, important for us as social animals, interaction with others.[5] For instance, your internal sleep/wakefulness cycles are synchronized with the external light exposures of day/night. Get too much light at the wrong time, and you'll have problems. We've all heard that we should avoid screen time before bed, and it's not to ruin our fun. Light directly interferes with our sleep, and research suggests that such late-night exposure might be linked to cancer, obesity, diabetes, and cardiovascular problems.[6]

Dr. Wendy Troxel, a senior behavioral and social scientist at the RAND Corporation, contends that partnered sleeping can help the body release zeitgebers and keep us in healthy rhythms. "Partners can be very helpful to help enforce consistent sleep and wake routines," she said. "It becomes a reminder to go to bed instead of staying up late playing video games or binging on Netflix."[7] Though Dr. Troxel concedes that many studies associate sleeping alone with a better night's sleep, those same studies reveal that people strongly prefer social sleeping. "Prioritize sleep as a couple. Think of it as an investment in your relationship, because you really are a better partner as well as more productive and healthier and happier when you sleep better," Dr. Troxel said.[8] Whether we opt for social or solitary sleep, we must ultimately curtail our late-night light exposure and develop other healthy sleep hygiene practices to keep our internal cycles harmonious.

You've probably heard of *circadian* rhythms, a Latin word meaning "about a day," which refers to our bodies' core endogenous rhythm. This twenty-four-hour internal clock is the same as the time it takes for the earth to rotate on its axis—a rhythm so fundamental that it has made its way into our genetic codes.[9] Your circadian rhythm coexists and moves in harmony with many (if not most) physiological and behavioral processes that occur, cyclically, every day of your life. These include your sleep/wake cycles, levels of alertness, body temperature fluctuations, blood pressure variations, reaction times, hormone secretions, digestion, and bowel movements.[10]

On a local level, many of these functions themselves run on shorter, recurring *ultradian* rhythms. Think of sleep, which happens in approximately ninety-minute cycles throughout the night. As it turns out, ultradian cycles of around ninety minutes operate during the daytime too.[11] Most of us can't maintain optimal productivity for over ninety minutes at a time, as our energy and creativity naturally ebb after such sustained focus. Instead of another cup of coffee, or disciplining yourself to keep your "nose to the grindstone," try taking a break after every hour and a half of work.[12] You might find yourself refreshed and recharged, ready for another ninety minutes of focused work.

Digestion, appetite, blinking, and sexual arousal also run on shorter rhythms. Some of these processes happen with precision and regularity. Others, like our hunger or the cycles of our moods, are more mysterious. Either way, these automatic processes tend to fade into the background as we go about our lives. We don't pay any real attention to them until they become disrupted in some way. And then, as we'll see, we frequently are forced to pay *a lot* of attention.

The Neuroscience of Rhythms

Have you heard about a "master clock" in humans and other mammals that helps to govern our rhythms and biological processes? It isn't simply a metaphor, but a real place in the brain's hypothalamus, located in a cluster of about twenty thousand nerve cells known as the suprachiasmatic nucleus (SCN). Situated right above the optic nerve, the SCN is sensitive to external stimuli, which help it keep accurate "time."[13]

In the absence of external zeitgebers, this master clock maintains a free-running rhythm of between twenty-four and twenty-five hours—your intrinsic circadian rhythm.[14] Because the shift from dark to light/light to dark happens twice per day, this synchronized rhythm is also called the *diurnal rhythm*. We synchronize ourselves to the daily rotation (rhythm) of the planet in step with our diurnal rhythms. But as I'll discuss later in the book, the way we behave in the modern world often disconnects us from this planetary synchrony. The diurnal rhythm becomes disrupted if our SCN receives a light signal when it is expecting darkness, or darkness when it is expecting light. We all know what it's like to feel groggy after a long flight—our diurnal rhythms are out of sync, and in conflict with external stimuli.[15] People who habitually reverse their natural diurnal habits, by working the night shift, for example, also experience disruptions in sleep and, as we'll see, are even more vulnerable to chronic diseases.[16]

You might have heard about the hormone melatonin and wonder how it fits into this rhythmic mix. When night falls, and our SCN no longer senses light, it signals the pineal gland to produce and release melatonin. As this hormone gets into the bloodstream, we become less alert, and the idea of sleep becomes much more enticing.[17] We've all been there! Melatonin is classically thought of as a sleep hormone, but as you will read later, it is perhaps best thought of as the *darkness* hormone. Our bodies release it in the absence of light, and for most of us, sleep happens to occur during this time.[18] You've likely seen it advertised in grocery market aisles and on Amazon—it's the only hormone authorized for sale without the need for a doctor's prescription.[19] Since melatonin is linked to the dark of night, the longer the night lasts—as it does through fall and winter—the longer our exposure to melatonin. Conversely, the long days and relative short nights of spring and summer shorten the duration of melatonin output released at night. (Unless, of course, we're popping the melatonin we've purchased from the pharmacy like they're breath mints!)

Melatonin, then, is the chemical messenger that links the expanding and contracting cycles of light in our external environment to our own master clock. Melatonin plays a role, for example, in synchronizing digestive secretions and enzyme pulses, as well as periods of immune system activity. Even your skin has its own diurnal rhythm, exhibiting greater resilience to UV radiation early in the day.[20] Melatonin allows the brain to orchestrate our seasonal rhythms and the biological processes that are best synchronized with these rhythms.[21] But when we expose ourselves to light at night, even in small amounts, melatonin production declines and all these processes become unaligned. Yes, that means that creature comforts like a night-light, and the innocent-looking light emissions from our electronics and consumer appliances, might be imperiling our sleep—and, by extension, our health. Small things can make big differences.

A Seasonal Model of Health

Our biological rhythms and the mechanisms by which they operate can become fairly complex when you get deeper into it—I've only just scratched the surface. But these rhythms become simpler, more intuitive, and more useful from the perspective of personal health when we look at them *experientially and behaviorally*, and in terms of the key hormones in our brains that help shape our experiences and behaviors. In the core areas of how we sleep, eat, move, and interact, we can break our experiences of sleep, food, movement, and social contact down into four conceptual blocks or seasons that occur throughout the year—spring, summer, fall, and winter. As a prelude to the rest of the book, let's take a quick look at each of these seasons in turn.

We start with spring. Within the context of the annual seasons, spring is the moment we start to become more physical, awakening from the slumber of winter. The coming of spring signals rebirth and reincarnation, which some people mark in religious traditions like Easter, and others in the annual "spring-cleaning" ritual of sprucing up the house. Many of us are titillated with the coming of spring, anticipating the fun and energy of summer that soon awaits.

Some of this titillation likely derives from spring's food offerings. In spring, there are fewer root vegetables and squashes left over from last fall, and the earth produces more fresh, fast-growing vegetables, like leafy greens. When I think of a hormone that best typifies this season,

I think of dopamine. Please understand: I'm not making a physiological argument about hormone thresholds correlated to each season. Instead, I've come to think of our calendar seasons as having personality traits and characteristics. Certain neurotransmitters and hormones, which are constantly coursing through our bodies, typify or embody essential elements of the different seasons in fascinating and sometimes uncanny ways. Take spring's dopamine. From a neurochemical standpoint, dopamine signals spring in that it triggers or motivates us to take risks, seek novelty, explore, become curious. Technically speaking, dopamine is a neurotransmitter, as it's released by brain cells called neurons. Dopamine, of course, is infamous for its role in reward, pleasure, emotional regulation, and addiction. Springtime is essentially the season of dopamine, and there's nothing wrong with that.

When it comes to seasons, spring and summer are thematically connected. They are both, broadly speaking, outward-looking, expansive, productive seasons. After we're done cleaning our houses, we're inclined to explore and meet new people and go new places in the spring, something that expands and intensifies during the months of summer parties and neighborhood barbecues. As spring develops into summer, our bodies crave more carbohydrate-rich, energy-dense foods. Sugary fruits are naturally plentiful during this period, and our ancestors gorged on them whenever possible. When I think of summer, the hormone that immediately comes to mind is adrenaline, a hormone that's well known for its role in responding to perceived stress. Adrenaline is useful because it helps us to focus and perform under that stress. And get this: adrenaline is biochemically made from dopamine.[22] Dopamine, which gets us jazzed about things to come, is biochemically converted into adrenaline, which helps us perform well and conquer the stressful challenge, however we might define these terms. I find it fascinating and even profound that the symbolic theme for spring (dopamine) is biochemically converted into the symbolic theme for summer (adrenaline). For our ancestors, performing might mean going into battle against a neighboring tribe or hungry predator. For modern man, it might mean summoning the courage to open your business or propose to your long-term partner. Either way, adrenaline is about *action and engagement*, and summer is all about performance and its subsequent stress.

During the summer, adrenaline courses throughout our bodies because we live in an extended period of stress—all of those late nights, all that stimulation, all the things to do, all that hard work. At this point, you might be thinking, "Hang on, Dallas. Summer is about relaxation and the beach. It's not stressful." I'm not talking about stress in a negative, psychological sense. I simply mean demands placed on the body and mind that require cognitive and metabolic resources. No doubt, dopamine and adrenaline both feel good. We even call thrill seekers "adrenaline junkies," a reference to the addictive properties of these endogenous substances. In fact, stress hormones and endorphins (natural painkillers), and all of the experiential hallmarks of spring and summer, feel *so* good that we have trouble moving away from them, even when it's no longer summertime. When we become hyperstimulated and overloaded, then we experience stress in a more negative and costly way. We become *stressed out* in the popular sense of being over-taxed, frayed, depleted.

The seasonal pivot from summer to fall is crucial and difficult to make. During the fall, fresh fruit supplies naturally dwindle, and the earth produces lower-sugar, starchy root vegetables. With cooler weather and shorter days, we tend to gravitate to heartier, meatier comfort foods. The Thanksgiving table is an ideal representation of what the fall diet is all about. A complete protein is the meal's centerpiece (the turkey), accompanied by hearty, satiating vegetables like mashed potatoes. There isn't typically kale salad with strawberries and feta cheese at the Thanksgiving table, unless you're trying to placate your vegetarian aunt from California. Tender greens and berries are *spring* fare, and at the Thanksgiving table they would seem out of place, as our bodies at this time of year naturally crave more protein and naturally occurring fats, with less emphasis placed on consuming sugar.

Now if what I said about kale salad in fall was hard to hear, prepare yourself because it gets even harder: this is a normal time to gain a little bit of weight. Think again of the stereotypical overeating we often see at Thanksgiving. It's conceptually consistent with the spirit of this transitional season, as our bodies are biologically saying, "I have to eat a bunch of calories because the cold winter is coming, and I really should prepare with putting on some extra body fat." This modest, seasonal weight gain isn't abnormal or at all damaging. The problem, once again, is when we get stuck in a certain mode and don't graduate to a different phase that would naturally rebalance the preceding seasons. When I think of autumn, the neurotransmitter that comes to mind is serotonin. Serotonin is associated with reward and pleasure, as well as meaning and gratitude. It's an adult version of adrenaline—it feels good, but still prompts us to think about the broader picture, about cooperating with others, and about the future. As I'll explain in more detail in later chapters, serotonin is also associated with leadership, with contribution to the community, and with connectedness to others.

Just like spring and summer, the phases of fall and winter are conceptually related to one another. While, generally speaking, the spring-summer block is largely about moving fast, working hard, and looking out for ourselves, fall and winter are seasons of slowing down, reconnection, and increased intimacy and generosity with the people who matter the most to us. When the winter months arrive, the natural carbohydrate availability recedes even more, and we incline to more dietary fat (with complete protein staying as a pretty consistent feature across all the seasons). This corresponds with a natural reduction in overall physical activity during these cold months, especially those that require large amounts of dietary carbohydrates to support (think hard running or cycling). We all know what comes to mind when we think of winter foods: short ribs, hearty and warming stews, and soup, something that will warm and nourish us after being out in the cold.

When I think of the interpersonal warmth and closeness associated with winter, I think of the hormone oxytocin. Fall's connectivity, characterized by serotonin, is a fitting precursor to the winter's oxytocin, a critical neuropeptide (something neurons use to communicate among themselves) that's crucial for strengthening deep and intimate bonds between people. Oxytocin is released during pregnancy, childbirth, and breastfeeding. It's been stereotyped as the "love hormone" because it is released during intimate romantic and sexual encounters as well, and even during conversational eye contact, close physical proximity, and nonsexual touch. So it's less the "love hormone" and more the "bonding hormone," which allows the broad connectivity of fall to yield to the deeper intimacy, trust, and closeness of winter.

Stuck on Summer

What a beautiful cycle. Our social interactions, activity, sleep, and nutritional inputs harmonize elegantly with the passage of the seasons. But, you probably guessed it, there's a problem. In the modern world, we've become like Kim: stuck on summer. By that I mean we become stuck in a world of (mostly) pleasurable stress. Summer, as we've seen, is a great time, both literally and metaphorically. It's a period of long days and short nights, brimming with activity and stimulation. It's when the neurochemical stimulation of hormones and neurotransmitters like dopamine lead us to gorge on sugary, carbohydrate-dense fruits. And that's biologically *normal* . . . in the seasonal context.

But following our organization into sedentary civilizations after the agricultural revolution (ca. 10,000 BC), we gradually abandoned any seasonal oscillations, and have had a hard time making the annual pivot to fall-type behavior. Once we started cultivating grain and other agricultural plants, carbohydrate-rich foods became available all year long and eventually formed the backbone of our "civilized" diets. Following the industrial revolution a few hundred years ago, highly processed, high glycemic index, sugary foodstuffs became continually available as well. As I said, it's normal for us to crave such foods when experiencing the stress of summer. Those cravings are appropriate responses to short-term stressors. Unfortunately, many of us never switch out of summer mode, meaning we live for years or even decades preferring and actually building our entire food system around the carbohydrate-centered diet of summer.

Many of our modern ills arise from our entrenchment in a perpetual summer mode. Take sleep, for example. When we expose ourselves to artificial lights in our office buildings, fluorescent lights in grocery stores, and the blue wavelength lights (such as those emitted by our phone and computer screens) that potently disrupt our normal circadian rhythms, we give our brains the message that it's daytime, and it's summertime. The quantity and quality of our sleep both suffer, causing our bodies to crave quick energy in the form of carbohydrates. Yes, disrupted circadian rhythms contribute to sugar cravings. When we're bathed in disruptive artificial light, especially after the sun has set, it becomes increasingly difficult to hear the deeply intuitive part of our bodies saying, "Hey, it's wintertime, go for the nourishing beef stew instead of the soda and chocolate muffin you're eyeing."

And that drowning out of intuition and satiety signaling leads us directly to overeating and obesity. When our rhythmic ancestors over-ate sugary fruits and seasonal plants, displacing some dietary fats and complete animal protein sources, it made sense because seasonal sum-mer stress made us neurochemically inclined to prefer energy dense, sugary foods over complete, more deeply satiating dietary proteins and healthy fat sources. But whole foods containing complete proteins and fats aren't just great to consume because they are nutrient dense—they are also the most satiating of the macronutrients, and as such they sup-press our natural hunger signals more effectively than the same number of calories from carbohydrates. Overeating carbohydrate-laden foods, especially carbohydrates from refined, low-nutrient sources, year upon year, leads to the dysregulation of our appetites and metabolism, set-ting us up for more cravings and overconsumption. Our bodies become chronically inflamed, metabolically deranged, overweight, and chroni-cally diseased as a result. A chronic summer diet causes chronic disease.

It's easy to get there because, let's face it, transitioning from summer to fall is hard. It's tough to tear ourselves away from the fun and frenzy of the summer's Las Vegas Strip and settle into autumn's quiet cabin in the woods. This makes sense intuitively and neurochemically: expan-sion and excitement is so much more neurochemically motivating and rewarding than contraction and restfulness. In today's world, summer is the expansive action phase, whereas the contraction phase requires more attentiveness and self-awareness to implement. In the natural world, it simply happens as a part of the whole cycle, but in today's world, we need to deliberately reintroduce contraction phases, as well as reframe contraction as balancing, stabilizing, and healthy. When's the last time you heard a positive news headline detailing how excited everyone was about a contracting stock market or smaller company earnings? Expansion is crucial. Think about what would have happened to our hunter-gatherer ancestors if they were not neurochemically motivated to explore, take risks, or seek novelty: they would have stayed in one safe and quiet place, depleted their resources, and probably starved to death. We needed the neurochemical motivation of dopamine and the performance enhancement of adrenaline to act, take risks, learn new things, explore the world . . . and survive. But problems arise when we don't confine such action to the appropriate season, or when we don't stop exploring. Like a seafaring explorer, we need to return home to port periodically, or else we're simply perpetually lost at sea, running low on supplies and feeling disconnected from our roots.

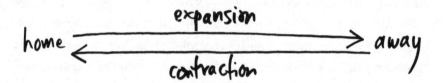

Let's not forget: while dopamine and adrenaline are pleasurable, they also cause us to become shortsighted and self-centered. They give us focus on the challenge or scenario at hand, but they also put blinders on us—blinders to other perspectives, other people, other ways of being. This is partly why drug addicts often lose track of practical aspects of their lives; they get hyperfocused on destructive neurochemical patterns. These neurochemical stimuli might feel amazing in the moment, but they don't lead us to plan wisely for the future or reflect deeply on the past. They don't facilitate broad, integrated thinking, or peaceful introspection. I don't know about you, but being stuck in summer is exhausting too. Don't you often feel like a lot of parents do at the end of the summer, wondering when the kids will go back to school so you can get a break? We often look forward to the fall for the shorter days, which mean earlier bedtimes. If that sounds familiar, you aren't alone. Many of us, myself included, have the perpetual sense of being frazzled and run-down, but we tell ourselves that we can't just stop in the middle of the madness (unless we get an illness, which is often the body's way of saying, "Hey, I really need some more caring attention over here!"). The feeling of being overextended is one that many of us carry for years and decades. You might not even recognize it anymore because you've lived with late summer exhaustion for so long. But if that's how you're feeling, take note: that's not okay. If it feels out of balance, that's because it is.

Breaking Free of Summer—and Getting in Tune

Many of us can at least partially identify with Kim's life—I know I have at various points in my life. Let's say that I only had an hour to consult with her. This is how I'd begin our journey together. I'd introduce her to the simple concept of expansion and contraction, of seasonal change, and encourage her to begin to develop a rotating or oscillating mind-set. When it comes to her social interactions, I'd encourage her to think of ways she and her family could slow down and be present with one another at some moments, while still pursuing activity and stimulation at others. Kim needn't do anything radical. She could start with simply spending more time with her kids, bracketing out some time to talk about everyone's day, or maybe even suggest meditating as a family. The larger point for her and for all of us is to jump right in and start experimenting—and not just with restoring rhythmicity to our social interactions, but to our eating, movement, and sleep as well. It doesn't matter where we begin. So long as we begin somewhere, we'll gradually become more aware of our innate patterns, and how to honor them.

The summer-to-fall pivot is a confronting, surprising, and even counterintuitive transition. But as I'm going to suggest in this book, although we might like the stimulation and fun of summer, we might also feel a little hollow or empty inside from always being in this mode. As a result, nudging ourselves back little by little to some fall and winter behavior can prove to be healing and deeply satisfying. Kim, for example, probably doesn't want to go to wine and cheese with the girls every week, because she's exhausted. She might not want to attend all her children's classmates' birthday parties, although she might feel subtle pressure to do so. Sometimes we gravitate to larger social events and welcome the opportunity to attend or host grand occasions. But we can only know if this is what we really want, and not simply ingrained routine or social expectation, when we slow down and check in with our innermost desires. When we give ourselves permission to slow down, contract, and connect more meaningfully, intimately, and vulnerably with a smaller circle of loved ones, we usually experience a degree of relief from the perceived expectations to do everything all the time.

Our lives and our bodies can be so much healthier and more fulfilled if we slow down, settle in, and fully immerse ourselves in the restorative phase of fall. The summer lights will still be there, beckoning, next year. But for now, take a long-overdue opportunity to rest and recharge. Over the next four chapters, we'll explore in more detail how we become stuck in summer in the four key domains of sleep, food, movement, and social interaction. We begin with an area that so many of us misunderstand and neglect in our 24/7, always-on, technologically saturated world: the need for an honest night's rest.

CHAPTER TWO

It Starts with Sleep

t Starts with Food. Or so I thought. I've presented over 150 seminars and written two books about food, including one with that very title. But as I relayed in the Introduction, my work on food really grew out of a broader perspective connected to the seasons and the earth, and entailing physiological, psychological, and emotional components. It was meant to provide a framework of scientifically sound principles, within which people could create their own more granular, nuanced versions of health and wellness. Food was an important starting point, but never the sole focus.

In fact, my approach to health and wellness has always been multifaceted. Early in my career, I practiced physical therapy for almost ten years, gradually expanding into strength and conditioning work, nutrition, and functional medicine. When I first encountered people like Kim, I began experimenting with different starting points to jump-start their lives. I sometimes began with strength training and cardiovascular conditioning, trying to improve overall health through better metabolic rates, muscle mass, and the like. I also tried stress management as a point of entry. But I rapidly figured out that food was the most practical and impactful starting point.

When we're "stuck in summer," our problems become muddled, confused, and sometimes a bit frustrating. Food can be a useful place to intervene because dietary changes can indeed rapidly improve a person's quality of life. Other lifestyle changes are crucial to optimal wellness, but their effects are more difficult to perceive and oftentimes imperceptible. Looking back, however, I think I might have overemphasized food's centrality, and underestimated that of sleep. As I coached clients and gave seminars, I saw that when people didn't prioritize sleep, it didn't matter how impressive their diets were—their health, overall, was subpar. Sleep certainly works in tandem with nutrition; dietary improvements can lead to significant, sometimes dramatic, improvements in sleep. But for our physical, emotional, mental, and social health, sleep is a key foundational element. In many cases, sleep *eclipses* food in importance. So, I hereby correct myself: optimal health really does start with sleep and the inherent rhythmicity that it is (or should be) built on.

Our National Sleep Recession

I remember being approached by a woman in her late twenties after a seminar a few years ago. Let's call her Jill. She loved high-intensity interval training (HIIT) workouts, which involve short spurts of highly strenuous activity like sprinting, heavy lifting, or kettlebell routines. Research suggests that such workouts build lean muscle mass, increase metabolism, and are more efficient at improving fitness than working out at lower intensities for longer periods of time.[1] Jill's enthusiasm for HIIT training was apparent—she did these strenuous workouts multiple times a day, six days a week. She was largely following a Whole30/Paleo diet, avoiding processed foods, artificial sugars, and grains, instead emphasizing healthy vegetables and complete protein sources. From her quick overview, however, it was clear to me that she was likely restricting her food intake too much.

Here's what was baffling about Jill. At a superficial glance, she was a lean, muscular woman. Many of her friends and passersby on the street admired her body, and used words like "badass" and "hardcore" to describe her. "Wow, you are so lean and cut," people would fawn, "you inspire me to get off my rear and work out more." But appearances were deceiving. When you took a closer look at Jill, she came off as tired, in the manner of someone who's just pulled an all-nighter. Powered by caffeine and sugar, and deprived of sleep, most people who've stayed up look a little rough and haggard. They have bags under their eyes and a subtle slump in their shoulders. Jill certainly looked that way. Her skin also bore many hallmarks of someone who engaged in excessive amounts of high-intensity exercise. It was graying a bit and becoming prematurely wrinkled. I'd seen this a lot in my endurance training clients. The chronic stress of such intense workouts leads to ongoing cortisol release throughout the system, causing structural breakdown in things like collagen that keep our face and skin looking youthful and healthy.

Like many competitive athletes I'd seen, Jill was prematurely aging herself. And not just superficially. Her hormones had become unbalanced and her menstrual cycle was irregular, which meant she had severe PMS symptoms that could have led to infertility. She also didn't feel good on a day-to-day basis and relied on stimulants to power through those long afternoons at work. Hardly the picture of optimal health.

When I asked her about her sleep, she seemed baffled: *"What has that got to do with anything?"* To get to her morning workout, she was rising before sunrise. She then returned to the gym during some of her lunch breaks, when she could get away, or in the evening. By the time she had finished and driven home and fixed a meal, it was already bedtime. Or it should have been. Jill had trouble falling asleep, and for good reason. Her intense workouts ramped up cortisol levels, putting her into a fight-or-flight state. From an evolutionary standpoint, such a state of readiness, hypervigilance, and stimulation was a perfect response when we needed to fend off hostile predators on the savannah, to run or fight for our lives. But it certainly isn't optimal for a body preparing for sleep, and it prevented Jill from sleeping as much or as well as she might have.

Even when confronted with these facts, Jill didn't want to talk about her sleep or caffeine consumption. She wanted to know how much lower she should take her carbohydrate intake because she was struggling to move some stubborn belly fat. This is again something I'd noticed among distance runners and triathletes (and other recreational athletes): their arms and legs are muscular, sinewy, and fairly lean. But if you look closely, they often have a little pouch around their middle, a classic hallmark of excess cortisol release over long periods of time. Jill was sure she needed a dietary fix because at ten to twelve workouts per week, she simply couldn't fit in any more training. Following her evening high-intensity training, she would often need a couple of hours to unwind, which she would spend under bright lights at home, either watching TV, surfing the web on her laptop, messaging friends on her phone, or, more typically, all the above in turn.

She was layering stimulation on top of stimulation—news of her friends, the dopamine surges from smartphone notifications, the melatonin-reducing blue light from the Netflix show she streamed on her tablet. She would, eventually, drag herself off to bed, or fall asleep among her humming devices, collapsing more from sheer exhaustion than restful repose. Feeling tired but wired, it would generally be some time around midnight before she was falling into what she described as a relatively light sleep, with her alarm set for 5:00 a.m., ready to start it all over again.

I wish I could say this was a rare and extreme example. But such stories are more common than you might think. The exact details vary—sometimes the story doesn't involve getting up so early for exercise, but for a daily commute. Still, the overarching pattern is generally the same. Modern civilization is suffering through a massive sleep recession, with the CDC reporting that over one-third of US citizens get less sleep than the recommended seven hours each night.[2] In the early twentieth century, this wasn't the case. Americans logged around nine hours.[3] But along came artificial light, revolutionizing our economies and our sleep routines. Following the introduction and eventual ubiquity of the light bulb in the twentieth century and the rise of individual LCD screens throughout the twenty-first, our sleep has steadily declined.[4] Now, we get up early and stay up late in a world that stays lit 24/7. The ethos of the city that never sleeps has spread to the entire modern world.

Many of us offer up similar reasons for burning the LEDs at both ends of the day. There are not enough hours in the day to do *all the things we want or need to do.* There's the daily commute, becoming ever greater as we choose to live farther away from our workplaces or are forced to for economic reasons, such as affordability of housing. Early in the morning or late at night might be the only space we get for *me time*, away from work or our often overstimulated kids. Our days and our time are so overscheduled that the moment anything extra falls in our lap, we need to *borrow* (read: steal) time from sleep. We routinely treat our sleep like a credit card in that we feel like we have money to spend, but in reality are barely keeping up the minimum payments.

Is it *really* that bad, though? After all, recent evidence challenges the notion that our preindustrial ancestral cousins slept more than we postmodern humans do, and that we should be sleeping from sundown to sunup *because that's how Paleo man slept*. UCLA researchers followed the sleep habits of three contemporary nonindustrial societies.[5] Studying the few remaining societies that live without access to electric light, they reasoned, may illuminate current sleep trends. Absent artificial light and digital technologies, do we sleep longer and better?

At first blush, the research appeared to indicate that these populations spent much more time sleeping than most people living in modern society—seven to eight and a half hours each night. However, further analysis of the data collected revealed that of this time in bed, only five and a half to seven hours was actually spent asleep. This is roughly comparable to modern postindustrial societies.[6]

This research generated many commentaries and interpretations, the most obvious being that we can all relax—that midnight to 5:30 a.m. sleep routine you have is in fact perfectly normal. "The argument has always been that modern life has reduced our sleep time below the amount our ancestors got, but our data indicates that this is a myth," said Jerome Siegel, leader of the research team and professor of psychiatry at UCLA's Semel Institute of Neuroscience and Human Behavior.[7] "I feel a lot less insecure about my own sleep habits after having found the trends we see here," echoed lead author Gandhi Yetish, a PhD candidate at the University of New Mexico.[8]

I can't quite embrace that conclusion. The sleep patterns of these tribes seem to work well for them, but based on my work with hundreds of consulting clients, that same amount of sleep doesn't seem to support healthy outcomes in different, more stressful environments. We industrialized humans burn the metaphorical candle at both ends . . . with a blowtorch. In the same way that doing a lot of intense exercise requires more nutritious food for full recovery, living a modern life of stress and overstimulation might require more sleep than if we were living like our electricity-free counterparts. Sleep of closer to eight or nine hours might be required if we're perpetually dealing with the sum total of financial stress, environmental toxins, inflammatory processed foods, social pressure to look a certain way or to acquire more material belongings, and chronic exposure to junk light (reducing the quality of our restoration during time spent in relative darkness, whether we're asleep or not).

Hello, Darkness, My Old Friend—and Hello, Light

One of the many major differences between the preindustrial societies the UCLA team studied and the sleeping habits of humans in modern societies is less about time in bed and more about the level and duration of *darkness* we experience before sleep.[9] To initiate the high-quality, restorative sleep we all seem to be craving, darkness is crucial. But darkness is something many of us only get once we are in bed and attempting to fall asleep. Even then, given the prevalence of bright alarm clocks, LED lights from the various devices in our bedrooms, light pollution from external sources such as streetlights and vehicles, not to mention both the light and sounds emanating from phone notifications coming in at all hours of the night ("but my phone is my alarm clock"), our supposedly dark bedrooms are anything but.

While many health experts rightly emphasize the importance of sleep, very few explicitly mention the biological importance of spending time in darkness before we get into bed. One exception is Richard G. "Bugs" Stevens, professor of medicine at the University of Connecticut, who was surprised that time spent in darkness wasn't a factor in the UCLA sleep study: ". . . a crucial aspect of the study's findings has not been discussed in news stories or the paper itself," he observed in the *Washington Post*. "People in preindustrial societies spend much more time in darkness than people in the industrialized world."[10] Yet it is becoming increasingly evident to specialists like Bugs that humans have a daytime physiology, triggered by bright natural light exposure, and a nighttime physiology, triggered by the absence of light and exposure to darkness.[11] In our daytime state we are (or should be) alert, active, productive, and hungry, driven by key daytime hormones and neurotransmitters such as cortisol, dopamine, and serotonin. After sunset, we transition to our nighttime physiology— our body temperature begins to fall, our metabolism slows, and our readiness and drive for sleep increases as the sleep hormone melatonin surges through our bodies. Except, as we saw in the last chapter, it isn't a sleep hormone, per se. It's a *darkness* hormone.

Come on, admit it. You sidle up to your laptop and watch *This Is Us* or random YouTube videos for an hour, bathing your eyes in artificial light. But then you get dozy, and finally turn off your television, smartphone, or computer, hoping that slumber quickly follows. Except it doesn't always, does it? That's because our daily rhythms are just like the seasonal ones—they require transitional periods. Our bodies are not like light bulbs that are either on or off. Every night, our bodies need to shift from one physiological state (daytime) to the other (nighttime). Absent this gradual transition, we remain restless, becoming progressively more anxious—often to the point that we can't fall asleep. And when we can't sleep, we indulge in still more screen time or we indulge in nighttime snacks, getting up to watch TV, have a bowl of ice cream, or scroll on our phone. Or we turn to sleep aids, from mechanical to herbal to pharmaceutical. In 2015 Americans spent $41 billion on white-noise machines, sleep-inducing mattresses, sleep coaches, sleep gadgets and smartphone apps, and other such paraphernalia. By 2020 a BBC Research analyst predicts that number will swell to $52 billion.[12]

So, what's the answer? Should we just turn out the lights after sunset and assume that we've solved our sleep-related maladies? I wish it were all that easy. First, if you think asking people to give up a favorite food and change their diet is hard, try prying their smartphones and tablets from their hands. Second, and most pertinent, the dark needs to be balanced with the light. Our nighttime physiology is inextricably linked to our daytime physiology, which itself is highly dependent on our exposures to sufficient bright light, particularly in the early morning.

And therein lies the rub. We're getting *too much* light at night, and we're also not getting *enough* bright light during the day. For many of us, perhaps most of us, our days and nights have become inverted. We are living in *dark days and bright nights*. I'm not just talking about night-shift workers here, though clearly this is the most extreme example. A significant portion of the population in our modern developed societies work indoors, where exposure to natural light is scarce. This includes retail workers deep inside multilevel shopping malls, office workers without a window seat, factory workers operating inside windowless buildings, medical staff working in hospitals, and air traffic controllers in blacked-out radar rooms. I recently observed that a local bicycle store permanently blacked out their windows (the only source of natural light) just to fractionally increase the shelving space inside by a few square feet. In addition, with the continual rise of urbanism and large sprawling cities where few can afford to live close to where they work, many people must leave home before sunrise and return home after sunset, for much of the year.

But it gets worse. Look around on a bright, sunny morning and you'll often see a significant number of people wearing sunglasses. You'll even see this on the not-so-sunny mornings, or in the subway. In heavily built-up cities, such as New York, the surrounding buildings can block much of the available sunlight and cast significant shadows. But you will still see people wearing sunglasses, blocking the light further still. In stark contrast to our preindustrial human ancestors, who would have awoken slightly before sunrise and who would have spent their mornings actively exposed to bright natural light (sans Ray-Bans), we modern humans might be lucky to get thirty to ninety minutes of bright light exposure during summer mornings, often filtered by sunglasses and/or UV-tinted windshields, before we scurry back indoors, missing out on not only the peak brightness of the day, but also a significant duration of bright light exposure.

To understand our (lack of) light exposure further, we need to understand a couple of measurements: *lumen* and *lux*. Lumen is a measurement of light intensity (brightness) taken at the source of the light itself. As light travels away from its source, it scatters into the surrounding area and its intensity changes. Think about a bright LED flashlight shining directly into your eyes versus being fifty feet from it. Lux takes the lumens of a light source and factors in the area over which the light spreads, giving an indication of how bright, for example, a light source is in a particular room.

To give you some scale and perspective on lux readings, the light on a clear day in the summer can exceed 100,000 lux; on a dark and cloudy day in the same outdoor space, it can be as low as 1,000 lux. Full daylight but indirect sunlight can measure 10,000 lux. At night, with a full moon, it would be less than 1 lux. Sunrise or sunset on a clear day is around 400 lux. Now let's compare these natural light scenarios to some typical artificial lighting. Bright office lighting comes in around 300 to 500 lux (comparable to sunset). An office hallway might be around 100 lux. A very brightly lit home living space might come in at a similar reading to the office but is more likely to be under 100 lux. That means that bright natural daylight is one hundred to one thousand times brighter than our typical indoor lighting. That's a huge difference.[13]

Linda Geddes, author of the book *Chasing the Sun: The Astonishing Science of Sunlight and How to Survive in a 24/7 World,* set about on an interesting light experiment in conjunction with sleep researchers from the University of Surrey (UK). Following the same argument that I make here, that our preindustrial ancestors lived and slept in tune with the light and dark cycles of the natural world, Geddes set about to live for four weeks with as little exposure to artificial light after sunset as practicably possible (in the context of having a career and family to manage). Part of her experiment involved measuring the intensity of her light exposure during the day.[14]

On one particular morning, sitting in the park after dropping her children off at school, Geddes measured the light intensity at 73,000 lux. She took another reading at her desk once she arrived in her office, 120 lux. That is, the light in the environment she would be exposed to for much of the day was about one-fifth of the light intensity she might get immediately after sunset, and only a tinier fraction of what she would get if she were outside. Even moving to a desk closer to a window where it was sunnier, the light intensity was 720 lux—still over one hundred times less than her light exposure in the park earlier that morning.

Across the duration of Geddes's four-week experiment, where she attempted to get more light exposure during the day, her average exposure between 7:30 a.m. and 6:00 p.m. was just under 400 lux in the first week of the experiment and as low as 180 lux in the second (but these were still increases from her preexperiment baseline of 128 lux). The experiment did take place in the middle of a UK winter when sunset occurred at 4:00 p.m. Nonetheless, the magnitude of the difference in light intensity between indoors and out is clear, being in the order of at least one hundred times less for the indoor environments, irrespective of the season.

Inspired by Geddes's experiment, I purchased a light meter from an electronics shop and began tracking the brightness of the light in the various settings I would find myself in on a daily basis. Without exception, and irrespective of the weather or cloud cover, outdoor light was always at least ten times brighter than the indoors, and more often one hundred times brighter. Early in the morning, the light in my house might be 100 lux, while outside at the same time, in indirect light, it was 1,000 lux. At my local café, it would be 300 to 400 lux seated indoors, and 30,000 to 40,000 lux seated outdoors. Conversely, at night, I recorded outdoor readings of less than 1 lux, while indoors, with the bright, blue-light-emitting artificial lights on, I would get around 200 lux. Switching the main lights off and using a low-wattage incandescent lamp brought the brightness down to under 10 lux.

As these experiments demonstrate, we're not getting the bright light we need during the day. As a result, we're confining ourselves to chronic summer sleep. We are in effect living in the weak winter light of the high latitudes during the day. Our indoor lives send the message to the light-sensitive part of our brains that it's dawn or dusk most of the time. With our increasing bright artificial (blue) light exposure after sundown, quite literally at the push of a button and flick of a switch, we switch to high-latitude summer light in our evenings. No wonder our brains don't know whether to be alert or asleep a lot of the time! We're sending really inconsistent and incoherent light signals. In the following chapters, we'll discuss how we're in perpetual summer mode when it comes to our diet, physical movements, and social interactions. Playing out summer sleep patterns throughout the entire year is just as unnatural and damaging to our health. Returning to the natural oscillation of the light/dark cycle on both a daily and seasonal basis is a vital and often overlooked route to better health and wellness.

It's All About the Neurology, Baby

How exactly does insufficient exposure on a regular basis to bright light or darkness disrupt our bodies' physiology? Let's take a closer look at the basics of our light biology and the circadian and diurnal rhythms mentioned earlier in the book. Natural daylight—light from the sun—contains the full spectrum of light, including invisible ultra-violet light at one end (which is involved with vitamin D production in the skin, tanning, and, when overexposed, sunburn) and invisible infrared light at the other (which gives us the sensation of warmth and heat). It is a specific segment of this spectrum—the shorter wavelength blue-light spectrum—that is involved in signaling and synchronizing our sleep-wake cycles. The presence of blue light stimulates our transition to daytime physiology and wakefulness; its absence, the transition to nighttime physiology and sleep. It is this diurnal light-dark cycle that sets the *endogenous circadian rhythm* described in chapter 1.

Receptors in our eyes (called intrinsically photosensitive retinal ganglion cells, or ipRGCs) that make up part of our circadian rhythm system contain a vitamin-A-derived protein pigment, melanopsin, that is sensitive to intense blue wavelength light, the kind we get from sunlight not long after sunrise.[15] When morning light stimulates these receptors, it activates neural pathways and hormonal responses that

color temperature
(in kelvins)

10,000	blue sky	blue
9,000		
8,000	LCD screens computer monitors	
7,000	cloudy sky (daylight)	
6,000	LEDs	white
5,000	midday sun fluorescent lights	
4,000		yellow
3,000	incandescent lights	
2,000	sunrise & sunset	orange
1,000	candlelight, firelight	red

help increase our wakefulness, alertness, and body temperature. The light literally wakes up and primes our body for the day. That light also suppresses melatonin. As the intensity of blue light declines toward the end of the day, being replaced, at first, by visible red light (such as is seen at sunset, or emitted by firelight), and eventually full darkness, melatonin secretion increases, initiating our sleep processes and helping us to, hopefully, fall asleep. A key part of our brain, the suprachiasmatic nucleus (SCN), or the *master body clock*, coordinates and synchronizes these light- and dark-triggered circadian rhythm events day after day. We are exquisitely tuned to the presence or absence of light, and we have very specific physiological responses to differing light triggers.

When it comes to sleep, many people focus on melatonin as our primary "sleep hormone" because of the association of low levels of melatonin and poor sleep architecture (the cyclical pattern during our sleeping hours). When you lie awake at night, or have restless sleep, low melatonin is usually a big part of that. This often leads us to hit up the local drugstore or Amazon.com in search of melatonin supplements, which we use as either an everyday sleep aid or to stave off jet lag when traveling. Melatonin, however, is most potent when produced as a downstream product of our daytime physiology, specifically, its precursor, serotonin.

The neurotransmitter serotonin, which I've described as characterizing the fall season, is important to us every day. It helps regulate our mood, appetite, memory and learning, and, you guessed it, sleep. Exposure to bright early morning natural light boosts serotonin production (in conjunction with the amino acid *tryptophan* and other vitamins and minerals consumed as part of a protein-rich breakfast), providing the raw materials for the melatonin required for our nighttime physiology.[16] The converse is also true. The *low melatonin leads to poor sleep* train of thought is an oversimplification. In fact, *low morning light exposure plus a low protein intake (leading to low tryptophan and cofactor intake) leads to low serotonin production, which leads to low melatonin production, which leads to poor sleep.* If we don't supply the building blocks and bright daytime light triggers for serotonin synthesis, we won't have adequate serotonin to convert into melatonin. You know that pleasantly relaxed, tired-but-not-frazzled feeling you have after a long day of hiking or playing at the beach? And you know how you often naturally want to head to bed fairly early on those days, maybe after sitting around a bonfire with your friends or family, and how you usually sleep really well that night? Yeah, that's the effect of lots of bright daytime light, lots of serotonin production, and lots of melatonin availability. That's the *normal* experience of the effect of natural light on your physiology. At the same time, we all now know that nighttime, blue-light screen time suppresses melatonin, so we could still undermine a perfectly good day of natural light exposure with *un*natural light after dark.[17] This is so common that experts have a name for it: light-induced melatonin suppression, or LIMS.

Melatonin's role in sleep is just the beginning. Melatonin performs a variety of functions in the body, making it indispensable for a long and healthy life. Melatonin has antioxidant properties, meaning it fends off damaging free radicals in our bodies, thus protecting us from a range of maladies, from migraines to deadly neurodegenerative disorders like Alzheimer's.[18] Melatonin also enhances our immune systems, and appears to be protective against a variety of cancers, especially breast and prostate cancer.[19] Melatonin receptors are present in many parts of the body, including the blood vessels, ovaries, and intestines. Melatonin appears to help regulate reproductive hormones in women through its interactions with the ovaries and pituitary gland. Melatonin even influences the timing, frequency, and duration of menstrual cycles. Melatonin, in nonhuman mammals at least, also helps to cue mating.

Serotonin is the daytime neurohormone, but don't think of it as the *functional* polar opposite to the nighttime melatonin. Cortisol plays that role. Like serotonin, cortisol production is stimulated by exposure to bright light such as sunlight and is the primary hormone for getting us awake and going in the morning.[20] It's healthy and normal to have elevated cortisol levels in the early to midmorning, but not beyond. We all require a strong, well-timed cortisol rhythm, where cortisol rises sharply from early in the morning (just prior to sunrise), peaks

around midmorning following bright sunlight exposure (while melatonin is low), then drops away over the remainder of the day and into
the evening (as melatonin begins to rise once again in the absence of
bright light). When the rhythmic interplay between cortisol and melatonin is disturbed in any way, particularly chronically, our bodies pay
a high price. We've already mentioned how *chronically elevated cortisol*
is disruptive, causing premature aging and visible belly fat deposits in
chronically stressed people, both sedentary folks and recreational athletes alike. Many aspects of modern life serve to elevate cortisol and/
or suppress melatonin at inappropriate times, be it many of the common low-calorie diets, badly timed and/or excessively long fasts, excessive exercise (think: Jill's excessive HIIT regimen), shift work (and
the associated circadian rhythm disruption), the stress of overscheduled lives, or even the anxiety of scrolling through social media, a common pre-bedtime routine for many (note: feeling pressured to project
the right image on social media, or trying to equal or surpass the projected images of others, isn't optimal for inducing a blissful nighttime
repose). Comparison isn't relaxing, and social media has a comparative
aspect programmed right into it. All of these things serve to elevate
cortisol as a part of our stress responses to life's daily pressures.

With a basic sense of the underlying neurology in place, we're now
in a much better position to understand the devastating impact that
a lack of daytime bright natural light exposure can have. Recent research has suggested that spending too much time in relatively low-
light rooms could be changing the way our brains process information
and impairing the growth of new neural connections. "Are Dim Lights
Making Us Dimmer?" read the headline of one report I reviewed.[21]
Our increasingly indoor lifestyles are also thought to be behind the
global nearsightedness (myopia) epidemic, where up to half of young
adults in the United States and Europe, and upward of 90 percent of

Asian teenagers are affected—a massive change from a half-century ago. The strongest environmental risk factor for this large-scale loss of visual acuity across our populations of teenagers and young adults: the lack of bright natural light exposure associated with being indoors most of the day.[22]

Perhaps the best example of the impact a lack of bright light exposure can have on our psychological health comes from looking at those who suffer from the winter blues: seasonal affective disorder (SAD) and its milder variant, subsyndromal seasonal affective disorder (SSAD). SAD/SSAD is a form of depression that's related to light changes in the seasons, most commonly autumn and winter, but is known to also occur in spring and early summer. There seems to be a clear link between light exposure and a change in our mood, outlook, and well-being.

We know that many animals change their behaviors in the winter months as the light wanes, with some going into complete hibernation. A decline in serotonin levels with the reduced light exposure (both duration and intensity) and a concomitant increase in daytime melatonin levels, often in conjunction with dietary factors such as an insufficient specific amino acid intake, is at the heart of the winter blues we can often feel ourselves slip into.[23] Living far from the equator appears to be a key risk factor for experiencing seasonal affective disorders, further supporting the suggestion that changes in natural light exposures are fueling this phenomenon. Indeed, in high-latitude regions such as Finland and Alaska, around one in ten people are affected by SAD, and one in four by SSAD.[24] Compare this to fewer than two in one hundred people in Florida.[25] Seasonal mood disorders are also more pronounced in regions that suffer cloudier winters, further reinforcing the notion that light plays a key role in our mood and feelings of well-being.

Symptoms of winter-onset SAD include low energy levels, tiredness, cravings for high-carbohydrate foods (driving increases in body fat), sleeping problems, difficulty in concentrating, feelings of hope-lessness or worthlessness, and suicidal ideation. Rather than depres-sion, summer-onset SAD, driven by excessive light exposure (such as might be experienced during the "white nights" of high-latitude countries in the summer months), is more likely to be character-ized by anxiety and mania. The easily overstimulated, hyperactive, and obsessive-compulsive tendencies that accompany summer-onset SAD are more commonly associated with unhealthy weight loss rather than weight gain.[26] These extremes give us insight into the effects of light—too little, too much, poorly timed—on our mood and behavior. While both winter- and summer-onset SAD may rep-resent extremes, most of us function and experience variances in our moods along a continuum of light exposures. It's hard not to observe that rates of depression and anxiety are increasing as our light and dark exposure patterns are perhaps at the most extreme they've ever been in human history.

Insufficient bright light exposure not only leads to low serotonin levels and poorly timed cortisol pulses, but as bright light exposure also catalyzes dopamine synthesis, a lack of well-timed bright natural light can also lead to low dopamine levels.[27] Dopamine is our moti-vation, pleasure, and mood neurotransmitter, and is part of a system all too readily hijacked by modern life. Think about the overabundance of drugs, alcohol, pornography, gambling, and processed food. What propels us to seek out sunlight, and what's responsible for the euphoric feelings we get once we are in it? Dopamine. Knowing this, it should also come as no surprise that shopping mall display lights are set signifi-cantly brighter than the lighting in other areas.

The symptoms of low dopamine include low mood, fatigue, apathy, a lack of motivation, an inability to concentrate, that "I can't be both-ered feeling," and cravings for highly rewarding foods containing sugar, fat, and salt. Reread the symptoms of winter-onset seasonal affective disorder above. Sound familiar?

Rediscovering the Dark Side—and the Light

For the vast majority of our evolutionary history, we have remained connected to and synchronized with the planet's natural light and dark oscillations, including the slow and steady ebb and flow of these cycles across the seasons. Despite the invention of the electric incandescent bulb, natural light and complete darkness still represent the two most powerful influences on our circadian biology. The consequences of our inverted light exposure are immense, traversing nearly every aspect of our biology. Yet most of us, most of the time, remain ignorant of the profound impact that light and darkness have on us. We resign ourselves to low mood, low energy, and bouts of anxiety and depression, because, well, that's just modern life. That's just the way it all is. But I don't buy that story.

By becoming more aware of the effect our light exposure patterns have on us, we can become unstuck in many areas of our life. For example, do you find yourself craving sugar, especially after dinner? By staying up late at night in the presence of artificial light, we give our bodies the message that it is daytime in the summer. This not only inhibits melatonin production, but it causes us to crave more sugar, as we're adapted to do during summer. But perhaps one of the surprising takeaways from this chapter is that a lack of early bright light exposure has the same effect. Experiment on yourself over a few weeks and see whether early light exposure influences your sugar cravings throughout the day. For those lucky few of you who don't have a sweet tooth, expose yourself to light and see whether you notice a difference in your energy or mood levels (indications you might have experienced more restful slumber). You can begin to develop self-awareness and intuition by simply asking, "How do I feel in the morning?" and reflecting on the response. You'll be better equipped to notice midafternoon energy slumps—perhaps as in Jill's case, addressed with sugar and caffeine— as well as anxiety and depression, both of which are linked with circadian dysregulation.

Whether we're trying to subdue our sugar cravings, increase our energy, rid ourselves of our abdominal fat, improve our mood, or get our lives and health "unstuck," we need to start with sleep. Become more aware of your sleep and light/dark cycles, and you'll find that your diet and physical activity levels will improve in concert, as will your emotional balance and natural connections with others. As kids, we might have been afraid of the dark. As adults, we're still afraid of the dark, but for a different reason: stuck on summer sleep patterns, we fear the lack of dopamine-releasing light indicating that someone has liked our Instagram status. We have the fear of missing out (FOMO), but that fear makes us treat our bodies in unhealthy ways. It's time that we paused to refamiliarize ourselves with nighttime darkness and daytime light, embracing the many health, longevity, and emotional benefits that come when light and darkness are in their natural balance. As best we can, we need to brighten our days and darken our nights.

CHAPTER THREE

Food Doesn't Have to Be So Hard

I s it just me, or are we all caught in a twilight zone of misinformation when it comes to food? First there was the low-fat diet push of the '90s and '00s, when everyone flocked to products like fat-free cookies and premade pancake mix with "low fat" proudly emblazoned on the packaging. Then, seemingly overnight, the ranks of the die-hard low-fat community diminished as new research suggested that all these hyper-processed low-fat foodstuffs caused sluggishness, heart disease, and pesky weight gain.

Not long after, the Paleo diet trend came and went. Premised on the notion that we should approximate the eating habits of our Paleolithic ancestors, this diet "Paleofied" and then commodified items like pasta and pancakes. A diet informed by our evolutionary history—that is, by our genetics—is the most logically sound starting point, but the movement failed to see the irony in rejecting modern bread, pasta, pancake mix, or cookie dough, only for its adherents to re-create gimmicky, supposedly "Paleo" versions of these same things. There's a huge difference between a whole-food, Paleo-type diet based on evolutionary principles and a modern, industrialized diet created with "Paleo" ingredients.

We now inhabit a confusing and murky post-Paleo world, in which some have turned to "plant-based" or vegan alternatives, and others have embraced low-carb or even ketogenic diets. (Ketogenic diets severely restrict carbohydrate and protein intake, relying primarily on dietary fat as an energy source.) What and how we eat has become increasingly polarized and tribal—a fact that should come as no surprise given our current political landscape. The world is increasingly contentious, and the diet world is no exception. For every diet guru, there's an anti-guru. For every early adopter, there's a skeptic telling you a given diet is a fad, unproven, and unsafe.

This turbulent food and nutrition environment, exacerbated by social media and marketing, causes a great deal of angst among health professionals. A friend of mine, a veteran naturopathic doctor specializing in women's health, strongly believes that women need nutrient-dense animal proteins—meat—for optimal health and function. (I couldn't agree more.) Yet after she was publicly vilified online for saying so, she steered away from discussing the topic at all. I know of other health professionals who consume meat, starches, vegetables, and salads but refrain from discussing it on social media for fear of attacks from online lynch mobs allied with particular diets. Read that last sentence again: people eating meat, starches, and vegetables fear social judgment. Crazy times we live in.

To be sure, food tribalism afflicts a relatively small portion of the world's human population that has the luxury of choosing its diet. Whether or not to blend Irish butter sourced from grass-fed cows into your Indonesian coffee is the epitome of a #firstworldproblem. But as we'll discover in this chapter, our *real* first-world dietary problems, which have now spread throughout most of the globe, are sources of widespread hardship and disease. Whether we eat a standard American diet or adhere to one of the healthier alternatives like unprocessed Paleo or intermittent fasting, we're still stuck on what I call chronic "summer eating" patterns. Since the agricultural revolution, when we flattened out our ancestral dietary oscillations, we've relied excessively on summer-style carbohydrates and long eating windows (eating early and late during our many waking hours). Abandoning food rhythmicity for continuous summer eating has produced chronic conditions like inflammation, insulin resistance, and obesity, and we all know that these things corrode our health and happiness.

How Our Ancestors Ate

For most of history, humanity has consumed diets that varied based on geographic location and available local food offerings. Our early human ancestors, who roamed the earth over two million years ago, were hunters and gatherers. Gradually, they fanned out from the equator, exposing themselves to a wide array of local foods. Certain societies ate a lot of protein and fat-rich nuts; others consumed large quantities of starchy root vegetables like sweet potatoes; still others ate whale blubber and very few carbohydrates. Then, around ten thousand to twelve thousand years ago, we collectively discovered that we could consume grass seeds (in other words, grain), and that by storing them properly we could stop migrating altogether and lead more stationary lives. We began growing grain, claiming ownership over the land to protect our annual crops. Giving up the hunter-gatherer lifestyle, we took up living in fixed settlements, choosing a narrower but less perishable range of food options.[1]

With a larger and more stable food supply and the ability to have more children (fueled by lots of easy carbohydrates), populations mushroomed and civilization progressed—we became better at language, developed rich cultures, and improved our survival rates. Agriculture powered such civilizational flowering, allowing us to produce more food and keep more people alive, at least long enough to give birth to the next generation. Agricultural foods began to account for ever greater shares of our caloric consumption, displacing the more varied sources of plant and animal nutrition we had enjoyed previously. Unfortunately, we are not well adapted to subsist primarily on cereal grains. They might increase our collective survival rates by allowing us to live long enough to reproduce, but they don't keep people resilient and healthy over our longer life spans.

Mummified remains in ancient Egypt and elsewhere bear witness to grain-based deficiencies like skeletal fragility, dental cavities, and maladies such as cardiovascular disease that were not widely present before the agricultural revolution.[2] And yet, we weren't about to give up on agriculture. As our sedentary ancestors expanded into towns and cities, population growth brought mounting pressure for more grain, further reinforcing our reliance on agriculture. With industrialization, our love affair with grain continued as we perfected the art of extracting the maximum amount of caloric energy from foods—much more than we need to enjoy optimal health.

From an evolutionary and ancestral health perspective, our diets shouldn't be based on carbohydrates year-round, as they typically are in modern civilization. Rather, our carbohydrate/fat/protein intakes should vary seasonally as our food selections vary seasonally. We've already observed how, during the warmer months of the year, our Paleolithic ancestors would have gorged on carbohydrates relative to dietary fats and complete proteins. This summer-type pattern of eating is roughly analogous to modern vegetarian, vegan, or plant-based (though not plant-exclusive) diets because it is higher in carbohydrates and somewhat lower in fat. But our ancestors didn't follow diet fads, and they ate both plants and animals year-round based on what was available to them. Instead, seasonal offerings dictated their higher-carbohydrate, lower-fat diets during the spring and summer seasons, as more relatively high-carb food sources—fruits, berries, honey— would have been more readily available for gathering. Consuming a large volume of nutrient-dense foods like these had metabolic and nutritional advantages during the warmer months. Naturally occurring fruits and vegetables are rich in antioxidants, which help protect our cells from damaging chemical compounds called "free radicals," which would be plentiful in our bodies during these months of summer stress. Compounds like polyphenols and carotenoids, which were abundant in these fresh plant foods, would have helped to protect our bodies from continual sun exposure and the oxidative stress of large amounts of physical activity.[3]

During the summer months, the accumulation of excess carbohydrates hopefully would have increased our body fat stores (and all of the summer's frenetic energy would have also improved our metabolic efficiency, aka fitness). This was important, given that carbohydrate-rich foods would have been in shorter supply during the fall and winter. As the air grew colder, the hunting of animals would likely have taken precedence over the gathering of plant foods (when's the last time you went berry picking in winter?). These animals, especially in the fall and early winter, would have carried greater amounts of body fat, skewing our nutritional consumption toward more complete proteins and higher fat. With higher-fat nuts and seeds also in greater supply, fall and especially winter diets would have likely contained moderate protein energy (10 to 35 percent of calories) plus relatively high-fat, low-carbohydrate, nonprotein energy.

Just like summer's antioxidants, winter's increased natural fat consumption would have conferred evolutionary and metabolic benefits. As we consumed more protein, and especially fat, we became more efficient at using fat for fuel, possibly even entering a special type of metabolic state called "ketosis." Ketosis requires the near-total absence of dietary carbohydrate and a huge amount of dietary fat, but some population groups who relied largely on animal foods in the winter would likely have moved into this adaptive metabolic scenario. An ancestral winter diet would have been somewhat analogous to the modern low-carb, high-fat or ketogenic dietary approaches, as well as to intermittent fasting protocols (given the relatively small daylight window that we had to gather and consume food in the winter). Going into winter ketosis would have helped us offset the metabolic effects of eating so many summer carbohydrates, while also allowing our bodies to experience flexibility in our metabolic pathways. That metabolic flexibility would have allowed us to stand a better chance of adapting to diverse nutritional environments. More adaptable organisms are better equipped to survive changing environments.

I have purposefully used terms like "relative" and "likely" throughout my cautious summary of hunter-gatherer eating patterns. Critics have attacked the Paleo diet movement and its offshoots for offering up simplistic narratives of ancestral life. I don't pretend to know everything our ancestors did and ate in great detail. My main point concerns the relative shifts in food consumption (and thus nutrient intake) that might have occurred over the seasons—perhaps only a few percentage points of energy intake in either direction. In the wider context of the seasonal environment, such smaller changes were substantial enough to alter downstream physiological processes. It would have been advantageous for our ancestors to utilize diverse metabolic pathways, enabling their bodies to thrive on antioxidant-rich, high-carbohydrate foods in one season, while using primarily fat to power their metabolisms in the colder months. That said, I don't wish to perpetuate Paleo fantasies and say this was *exactly* how our ancestors ate—we simply lack the historical evidence to make definitive claims. My point is that for most of human history, in most parts of the world, and in most cultures, our diets varied seasonally, oscillating just as our seasonal sleep patterns, modes of social interaction, and movement patterns did, and that we would all be better off if we honored some of the historical rhythms that our bodies expect.

The Good and Bad of "Fad" Diets

In other books, I've extracted lessons from this brief sketch of civilization and the flattening of diverse eating patterns, suggesting which foods we should eat and which we should avoid. Let's now take the discussion a step further and address larger lessons about how and in what context we should eat. I've gently criticized the Paleo, keto, vegan, and other plant-based protocols for their faddishness or lack of sound supportive research. Although these diets may not be optimal for our long-term health, they can all confer benefits over the short term for one simple reason: all of them serve to dislodge us from something much worse—the mainstream, highly processed, grain-based diet on which most of us are stuck.

Nutritionists call this mainstream approach to eating the standard American diet, or SAD. Given the ultra-processed Frankenfoods that feature prominently in this diet, SAD couldn't be more apt. In inflammatory, nutrient-poor pseudo-foods like cookies, chips, and microwave dinners, industrial processing has done all the hard digestive work for us, leaving us with food products that are effectively predigested (they've had their cellular structure largely removed or heavily altered), soft (don't require a lot of chewing, or worse, are in liquid form), and extremely energy-dense (contain fats and sugars in amounts well beyond what humans would normally consume). The presence of this excess energy, combined with the inability of this Frankenfood to suppress our hunger and truly satisfy us, leads us to regularly overeat and store the excess energy as fat. These so-called "foods" deliver us calories for survival, but they don't nourish us in a deep, satiating way. By leaving us without an intrinsic sense of rhythmic eating or of deep nourishment, they induce us to follow our stress-driven and reward pathways for carbohydrates, and especially sugar.

Veganism, vegetarianism, and other plant-based diets represent a marked improvement over the standard American diet. By prompting us to avoid or minimize animal protein, these diets boost the amount of whole-plant food a person consumes, increasing the share of nutrients we consume and improving our gut health. Like standard American diets, however, plant-based diets allow people to survive, but not necessarily to thrive. That's because plant-based diets make it difficult for us to meet our complete dietary protein needs. Once again, context matters. If you aren't physically active, a plant-based diet might give you enough protein. But plant-based diets tend to rely heavily on cereal grains and legumes, either because they're convenient and inexpensive or because they deliver some dietary protein.

Most of us were raised to believe that whole grains are important pillars in our diet, furnishing "complex carbohydrates" to power us through a workout or an afternoon at the office. Unfortunately, beans, lentils, barley, wheat, and rye—not to mention pizza, pasta, and bread—are nutrient-poor foods that contain various and often problematic compounds like lectins that inhibit nutrient absorption and proper digestion, and can cause inflammation in the gut. Additionally, foods like barley, wheat, and rye contain a type of protein called gluten that can cause intestinal problems and inflammation. Such symptoms can be severely detrimental to people with celiac disease or non-celiac gluten sensitivity, but they likely inflict some degree of damage on most of us, increasing systemic inflammation.[4]

Eating low-fat vegetables and fruit all year long sounds healthy and virtuous, but this summer diet is a poor selection in midwinter, when the chilling winds, ice, and snow (as well as the larger number of hours of darkness) leave us wanting something heartier, which typically means warm and calorie dense. In the winter, we don't require as many antioxidant-rich fresh plant foods, and naturally gravitate toward the higher-fat foods and complete proteins that help improve our ability to use fat as a fuel source. Not to mention: if you have snow on the ground where you live, that fruit and arugula would have racked up significant miles getting to you from warmer climes, decreasing their nutritional potency and placing undue strain on the physical environment. Bottom line: I want you to be strong, robust, and resilient, and I therefore can't recommend permanent plant-based eating.

As this book goes to press, low-carb and the more extreme ketogenic diets have surged in popularity. Although some research supports the metabolic merits of ketogenic eating, many people come to it simply because our conventional dietary approaches are failing, and they're desperately seeking alternatives. Carb restriction addresses our society's endless summer diet that overemphasizes carbohydrates and causes insulin resistance, chronic inflammation, excessive deposition of body fats, and other diseases of civilization. Instead of eating too many carbs, low-carb or keto diets will have us veer to the opposite extreme, sticking to the protein and fats that approximate what our ancestors ate in the fall or winter months.

Ketogenic diets consist mainly of healthy dietary fats, like avocados, nuts, and fatty animal proteins, while keeping protein intake moderate and carbohydrate consumption to an absolute minimum. Keto's underlying rationale is sound because when we perpetually supply carbohydrates, our bodies predominantly burn glucose (sugar), and if we limit carbohydrate and protein (some of which can be converted into glucose), our bodies will adapt and get considerably more efficient at using fat as a fuel source, including producing some special molecules called "ketone bodies" that our brains can use as a partial fuel source too. By abandoning chronic summer's carbohydrates, ketogenic dieters have unknowingly reaped the metabolic benefits of moving into a different season. They've abandoned endless summer and embraced the more stark and wondrous beauty of winter. A ketogenic diet is effectively a corrective strategy. But like plant-based diets, carb-restricted or ultra-low-carb ketogenic diets are not optimal ways to eat long-term. They are ideal for winter—and winter only. See the pattern here? Different seasonal modes of eating confer different benefits, all in their correct time, but none of them are truly optimal as a fixed way of eating long-term.

Something similar holds for another popular dietary approach, intermittent fasting. In the ancient past, we mostly ate when it was light out because the food we hunted and foraged was visible. The time convenient for us to eat varied seasonally as well. In the summertime, when we would rise early and retire late, we had many hours to chow down. In the winter, the shorter days narrowed our feeding windows. So once again, given the prevalence of chronic summer habits, it makes sense that people seeking solutions to chronic summer's harm might gravitate to fasting protocols. When people restrict their feeding windows (the hours that they choose to eat within), they move away from summer's very wide feeding window. Like low-carb/ketogenic approaches, such a lifestyle is corrective—an unwitting nod to our long-neglected winter eating patterns. Yet problems arise when we take the very wide feeding window of summer, or the very reduced one of winter, and apply it every month of every year for decades. That merely substitutes endless winter eating for chronic summer. We should oscillate in and out of both patterns over the course of the year. Both are good.

Unfortunately, many people embark on fasting protocols out of season. They usually start over the spring or summer months (often to get lean or "beach ready"), even though fasting is better suited to winter, with its naturally shorter days and the shorter eating windows they gave our hunter-gatherer ancestors. Among habitual fasters I've also observed a tendency to delay eating after waking and not break the fast until much later in the day, often after midday (something referred to as late time-restricted feeding). As we'll explore below, this strategy defies research suggesting that early time-restricted feeding (eating early in the morning, and fasting later in the day) is superior in terms of metabolic benefits.

If you search for any of these diets on social media, you'll see countless people testifying to their wonders. These diets have lowered fasting blood sugar levels, helped reverse diabetes, cleared up acne, and even helped people manage chronic pain. They've given people more energy and an emotional kick start, enabling them to leave toxic relationships, open new businesses, or approach life with more zest. But if we were to conduct further investigation, we'd likely discover that these diets worked well *for a season or two*. The benefits of these adaptations don't last indefinitely.

People aren't as inclined to post dramatic confessions about how their dietary choices have failed to produce results after an initial success. This lack of long-term "results" often leads people to shift strategies, or to double down on their current strategy, potentially leading them farther down a maladaptive path. If, for example, your low-carb diet isn't working as you'd hoped (perhaps because it's the right diet at the wrong time), you might decide to intensify your efforts by going even lower carbohydrate, or perhaps keto.

Keto does its best work as a corrective counterpoint to chronic summer, in which we constantly consume and crave. If we can manage to resist all of those tempting carbohydrates on offer in modern society, and instead consume almost exclusively fats and some protein, our bodies go into ketosis, which means they begin burning fat and ketones, instead of glucose, for energy. Ketosis represents a significant break from our glucose-driven chronic summer eating patterns. The problem, of course, is that dieters who see benefits on ketogenic diets conclude that keto is a permanent, year-round solution. Many online forums feature people measuring their ketone levels by urinating on ketone strips, fretting about the concentrations of ketones in their blood, and whether that chicken breast with lunch kicked them out of ketosis (rendering them a dreaded "glucose burner" again). Before you know it, people are afraid to eat even healthy foods and become more restrictive as their health begins to deteriorate.

Popular Diets: More Similar than Different?

Such anxiety is really a shame because, upon closer examination, all of these diets converge on a similar pattern. Take, for example, a healthy low-carb meal. What does that look like on a plate? Probably something along the lines of a hand-sized portion of protein plus some non-starchy vegetables. In such a meal the total carbohydrate is low, but the total fat may be higher (or at least higher than has been recommended over recent years). How about a healthy Paleo meal? On the plate, such a meal will represent something like a hand-sized portion of protein (typically animal protein) plus some nonstarchy vegetables. It may also contain some starchy root vegetables, but it is still likely to be lower in total carbohydrates than a typical Western or standard American diet meal. A keto diet? A higher-fat, very low-carb variant of the low-carb meat and vegetables. A vegan diet? If done right, plant-based protein sources plus vegetables. Carnivore diet? Protein sans vegetables. The Mediterranean diet? Protein with an emphasis on fish over red meat, plus vegetables. Intermittent fasting? When you do eat, you are encouraged to eat a good source of protein plus vegetables. Even the best versions of the old-school low-fat diets were . . . wait for it . . . protein plus vegetables. Think skinless chicken breasts plus steamed broccoli.

In addition to being similar, all of these diets boast similar benefits. In consuming whole foods instead of the preprocessed staples of the standard American diet, our digestive systems must work hard to break down cellular structures in order to extract a food's nutritional value (from the chewing and grinding of our teeth, to the acid bath of our stomach, to the enzymatic breakdown in our intestine). Such exertion limits the resulting payload of amino acids, fatty acids, and sugars entering our bloodstream, with the process taking enough time so that our hunger can naturally subside as we experience "satiation" (the desire to no longer eat). These diets also help promote a healthy gut microbiome. The human "microbiome" refers to the microbes, like bacteria, fungi, and yeasts, that inhabit our gut and help us do everything from regulate our immune system to metabolize food.[5] The concentrated fats and sugars contained in processed foods not only overwhelm our system directly, but they also skew the balance of our microbiome. But improving the gut microbiome can help reduce cancer, obesity, cognitive problems, and metabolic dysregulation.[6]

Although we have much to learn about the nature of the microbiome, shifting our eating away from processed food products and toward whole foods serves to drain the swamp. It decreases the numbers and types of bacteria that may, for example, promote inflammation in the gut, and creates a better balance of more desirable types that work more in concert with our immune system. Conventional dietary recommendations suggest we should consume more fiber in our diet, but I believe that "fiber" is just a proxy for the consumption of whole foods, of plant or animal origin, that have their original cellular structure either fully or mostly intact at the time we begin to ingest them. Consuming such whole foods improves both our gut health and total body wellness, given the important symbiotic relationship between human beings and their microbiomes.

Although the popular diets I've mentioned reduce the amount of ultra-processed foods we're eating and help improve our gut microbiome populations, they bring a number of disadvantages. Far too often, such diets, and the dietary tribes to which they give rise, define themselves in negative terms—emphasizing what they're restricting. If you're on any form of low-carb diet, your identity is carbohydrate restriction. If you eat a low-fat diet, you're all about fat restriction. If you eat a plant-based or vegan diet, your dietary identity centers on animal protein elimination. If you're an intermittent faster, you restrict a range of food but *not* during certain windows of time. These diet camps, in turn, believe that those failing to adopt their respective restrictions will experience dire health outcomes. The plant-based tribes say: eating too much protein or too many calories will shorten your life span. The keto enthusiasts claim that eating carbs produces toxic by-products, so we must restrict all sugar. The intermittent fasters say making our bodies constantly metabolize food diverts our organs from performing other vital tasks, so we must eat less often. Popular nutritional frameworks have become a fearmongering case of "restrict (something) or die."

Conversely, advocates of these diets often attribute their success to whatever restriction the individual or group embraces. A low-fat diet that cuts out cakes, bagels, muffins, and many other calorie-dense, ultra-processed foods, and replaces them with protein and fiber-rich plants, supposedly works because it reduces an individual's caloric intake by reducing the macronutrient with the highest calorie load—fat. Low-carb diets also work, the logic goes, because as carbohydrate calories reduce, so do insulin loads, promoting fat-burning rather than fat storage. Paleo works because it cuts processed grains, sugars, and fats. Veganism (again, when done well) also removes many processed foods (because such foods often contain ingredients such as milk or butter). No matter what diet we champion, we'll generally fly the flag for that diet based on what it primarily limits.

Still, each diet essentially represents a short-term, partial solution to chronic summer—an oscillation away from chronic sugar and carbohydrate intake to either a more moderate or "winter" mode of eating. This is the fundamental problem with the diet industry. It proposes short-term approaches that people interpret as global, permanent "solutions." In reality, these diets happen to provide partial corrective strategies that compensate for our chronic summer eating.

Eat Seasonally to Get More Protein

For the last decade of my life, and following numerous "what do you eat?" requests, I've defined my own eating with the following sixty-second elevator pitch, emphasizing seasonal oscillation:

I eat naturally occurring and minimally processed foods like meats, eggs, vegetables, and fruits. I choose these whole, nutrient-dense foods over packaged, processed foods, which are often nutrient poor but calo-rie dense. Food quality is important to me—a concept that includes where my food comes from (local), how it was raised or grown (humanely; organic), and what its overall environmental impact is. I aim for well-balanced nutrition, so I eat a diet of predominantly unprocessed plant-based foods, anchored by appropriate amounts of quality animal-based protein foods. This balanced combination of plants and animals provides me with all the nutrients I need, including all the proteins, carbohy-drates, and fats naturally inherent in these food groups. How I eat—the social and cultural aspects of food and nutrition—is just as important to me as what I eat.[7]

I deliberately crafted this pitch to show a very inclusive diet, and to signal that I make conscious decisions regarding the likes of ani-mal welfare, as well as the environmental, social, and cultural impacts of my food choices. In fairness, I restrict as well, as I generally avoid ultra-processed and processed foods. Such foods negatively impact my health, and because they contain cheaply made foodstuffs (like corn de-rivatives), lack local color and cultural significance, and reach my table after long voyages around the world, they also diminish our larger en-vironmental and cultural health. Despite my best intentions to convey a broad and varied diet, people still often label my way of eating as re-strictive, be it restricting carbohydrates (because I don't eat processed carbohydrate sources like pasta) or restricting fat (because I don't eat or drink "fat bombs" that are popular on the keto diet). The framing of such restriction usually depends on a person's own dietary bias. People typically want me to be their dietary ally or enemy (in the latter case, usually so they can pick a food fight with me). I've also been accused of not restricting my diet enough. I've been told that I could not possibly care for animals or the environment because I consume animal protein.

Somewhat perversely, by discouraging the consumption of highly processed packaged foods, I've also been accused of promoting disordered eating patterns.

To critics, I would point out that two important components of my personal dietary approach—protein and food timing—are often lost in nutrition discussions today. No matter our dietary tribe or philosophy, when talking food and nutrition, it's relatively easy to focus on fats and carbohydrates, our prime nonprotein energy sources. (Alcohol is the third source here and is typically the one most people don't want to discuss, a discussion we'll save for another time.) There is a tendency, in the nutrition community's long-winded and myopic debates, to either skip over protein or to dismiss it entirely. This is largely because protein energy constitutes a relatively small percentage of our total energy intake compared to the other two macronutrients. Warring dietary factions debate the merits of carbohydrates versus fat, as protein gets lost in the shuffle. Also, protein intake has remained relatively stable during the obesity epidemic's unfolding, and so hasn't triggered significant interest from researchers, clinicians, and practitioners.

There is, however, a growing body of research indicating that the amount of energy we obtain from protein determines our total caloric intake. The Protein Leverage Hypothesis, as this theory is known among experts, which has been corroborated by a substantial body of evidence, suggests that metabolically healthy humans actively regulate their macronutrient intake, and in so doing, prioritize protein energy over nonprotein energy (fat, carbohydrate, alcohol).[8] If our diet contains low absolute amounts of protein (and perhaps even specific amino acids from which proteins are synthesized), our appetites increase as an attempt to get us to seek more nutrients (including proteins), leading to the overconsumption of nonprotein energy as we attempt to fulfill our protein energy needs.

In other words, our protein requirements are such that we continue to eat until we reach our target protein intake, at which point our appetite and hunger subside. We'll eat whatever is around until we get enough protein. But in a world where the cheapest, most readily accessible foods are generally low in protein, or the protein they contain is not readily digestible and absorbable (such as wheat proteins), we often struggle to hit that target, in the process overconsuming nonprotein calories. In a review of thirty-eight published experimental trials measuring how much protein people consumed when they could eat as much as they wanted, total protein intake was inversely related to total calories consumed. The greater the amount of protein people ate, the less total energy they consumed, regardless of their fat and carbohydrate intake.[9]

A 2011 University of Sydney study tested subjects on diets containing either 10, 15, or 25 percent energy from protein. The results showed that lowering the protein energy from 15 to 10 percent significantly increased the total energy (made up of nonprotein energy) people consumed, primarily because they were snacking between meals.[10] The quality and composition of those snack foods? Processed foods rich in sugars, refined carbohydrate flours, and inflammatory industrial seed oils ("vegetable oils"). The trend is clear: if we consume less protein, we tend to increase our nonprotein energy intake, something that may predispose us to chronic overconsumption.[11]

Many health authorities don't know about this research and continue to recommend lower amounts of protein energy intake, primarily to limit meat consumption. That makes sense, particularly as the world grows sensitive to the impacts of agricultural greenhouse gas emissions and climate change. But pushing people toward lower-quality plant-based proteins, such as those from wheat or legumes, and lower amounts of protein in general, seems counterproductive if it results in more hungry people who will overconsume nonprotein energy to quell that hunger. If we truly worry about our global carbon footprint and feeding the world's ever-growing population, we should start limiting low-nutrient, nonessential foods first. Australian research estimates that about 27 percent of the food-related greenhouse gas emission footprint in that country comes from the production and consumption of "noncore" foods (fast food, candies, and the like).[12] In North America, this number is probably much higher. Demonizing high-quality protein foods leads to higher junk food consumption, ultimately compromising human health and the environment.

Consider the experience of Sarah, a client of mine. A busy young twentysomething, Sarah began most days with a standard bowl of cereal and milk before leaving for work. She wasn't much of a morning person, so she slept in as late as possible. By the time she showered, dressed, and did her hair and makeup, she had exactly three minutes and forty-seven seconds to eat breakfast before running out the door in a flustered rush. Not long after arriving at work, Sarah started to feel a bit hungry and contemplated what she would have at her midmorning break. If she was "being good," she would grab a piece of fruit, or maybe a low-fat yogurt. More often than not, she craved something a bit sweeter, and a nearby coffee shop was always happy to oblige. She ate lunch a few hours after this sugary snack, usually just a salad or a sandwich, sometimes a juice, but nothing particularly substantial.

By early afternoon, Sarah's appetite would explode. Having endured the postlunch energy dip, when she struggled to keep her eyes open and focus, her appetite would kick in aggressively. Quite often Sarah would claw at the office vending machine in a frenzied state of "hangriness" (hungry + angry), unable to decide if she wanted something sweet, savory, or both.

Arriving home late, tired, and hungry (again), Sarah would often eat a large meal, certainly her largest of the day—anything from take-out Mexican, Thai, or Indian that she picked up on the way home to a frozen pizza or mac 'n' cheese meal. Either way, dinner was usually heavy on the carbs (mostly from rice or pasta) and meager on protein.

Because Sarah ate little to no quality protein throughout the day, she usually got hungrier as the day progressed. The appetite center in her brain continually prompted her, in vain, to seek foods that might satisfy the protein her body desperately needed. In the absence of sourcing this protein from her diet, Sarah's body likely harvested it from the only real reservoir of protein in her body: her muscles and connective tissues. Meanwhile, she always thought about food, scrolling through Instagram's "food porn" photos, and asking friends and colleagues what they planned to have for dinner that night. Because of her workplace's physical and social food environment, and because she always felt stressed and rushed, she made consistently poor food choices.

Research suggests that the distribution of protein across the day is as important as the overall amount. The protein Sarah did consume was typically compressed into one meal and drowned out with foods (high-carb, high-sugar, and salty foods in particular) that blunted the satiety signal that protein typically provides. In general, it is better to eat three thirty-gram protein meals spread evenly across the day than a ten-gram protein meal at breakfast, a twenty-gram protein meal for lunch, and a large sixty-gram protein meal for dinner. The even distribution across three meals is also better than multiple, ten-gram "grazing"-type meals spread over the day. The smaller protein amounts aren't enough to trigger proper satiety levels, and so it becomes too easy to overconsume nonprotein energy across the day.

The large protein-rich dinners typical of North American society has led to the oft-repeated narrative that everyone already eats too much protein. If you were to focus on just one meal of the day, examine the total protein content of that meal, and ignore the satiety-disrupting effects of the highly processed sugars, carbs, fats, and salt that normally sit alongside this protein (think: a couple of burgers, fries, and cola), it is easy to arrive at this conclusion. In fact, many individuals under-consume high-quality protein, fail to distribute it evenly across the day, and, obeying their own powerful hunger signals (and/or lack of satiety signaling), overconsume nonprotein energy. It's high time we shine a light on protein and give it pride of place within our oscillating dietary framework.

Watch *When* You Eat

The problems associated with the common eating patterns of the near-globalized standard American diet aren't limited to the macronutrients we eat, like protein. We must also look at when we eat, as well as our context for eating. Many people mistakenly regard food simply as fuel, nothing more than calories and micronutrients to be balanced, varied, and moderated. But alongside nourishment, food also provides our body with information about the environment, synchronizes us with the days and seasons, and, more important, binds us to one another and to the physical environment from which that food derives.

When it comes to our circadian rhythm, food and eating, much like light, can be a powerful zeitgeber—an external environmental cue that helps to govern our natural rhythms, both those pertaining to the twenty-four-hour light/dark cycle and those related to the seasonal changes over a year. Without such external cues, our body's master clock (which itself "free-runs" over a slightly longer time period than the twenty-four-hour rotation of the earth) would progressively disconnect from the natural light/dark cycle of the local environments we inhabit.

We've observed how the light and dark signals of sunrise and sunset help set our circadian rhythm, and how insufficient and excessive bright light during the day disturb these rhythms. But other regular features of our days also help to synchronize and maintain this rhythm, including eating meals at regular times *during daylight hours*. Those last three words are key. Although modern society has normalized eating well into the night, such late evening feeding likely impairs our metabolic health and promotes weight gain, even when eating an otherwise balanced diet. *When* we eat matters a lot more than most of us recognize.

Research on eating and circadian rhythm biology at the Salk Institute found that human metabolic health—everything from the physical motility of our digestive system, enzyme release, and hormonal profiles in response to eating—is best when we confine eating to an eight-to-twelve-hour window, starting in the early morning and ending in early evening (relative to sunrise and sunset).[13] In research circles, this pattern is called "early time-restricted feeding."[14] When examining modern, real-world patterns, however, the same research group found that the average person eats over a fifteen-hour (or longer) period each day, often grazing on foods and drinks high in sugar, fat, salt, and, oftentimes, alcohol.[15]

Leaving aside the qualitative aspects of the foods and drinks we consume over such an extended period, consuming what is often the largest part of our total energy intake for the day over the period spanning late afternoon to just prior to bedtime (and sometimes even waking up in the night to eat) conflicts with our fundamental physiology. Recall from earlier in this book that we have a distinct nighttime physiology. Under the influence of melatonin, our bodily processes slow down, preparing us for the tissue and organ repair that accompany sleep. Under these conditions, our bodies simply can't deal with an onslaught of calories to process. Forcing them to do so leads to a variety of negative health consequences.

Consider glucose. You can think of glucose as operating in the opposite fashion as melatonin. The early daylight suppresses melatonin production, which only kicks in in a big way—ideally—at dusk, when the absence of natural light cues the secretion of the darkness hormone. The glucose coursing through our bodies follows an opposite pattern, gradually decreasing as the day wears on. The research is unambiguous: our bodies handle glucose better earlier in the day than in the evening or night.[16] Eating large meals at night (or many smaller meals combined with extended snacking), especially those rich in carbohydrates, can lead to increased circulating glucose (and increased insulin) at a time when the body's ability to healthfully and easily deal with both is impaired. In experiments where food intake is matched across subjects and only the timing of the meals changes (early morning versus late evening), subjects eating later in the day experienced higher blood pressure, worse blood glucose control, and increased body fat. Such changes, played out day after day, serve as precursors to the likes of cardiovascular disease, diabetes, and some cancers.

Just as our brain's master clock governs our physiology in response to light and dark signals, each of our internal organs comes equipped with its own internal clock (synchronized with the master clock) that regulates its daily cycle of activity. Within the gut, this clock controls everything from the flow of digestive enzymes and stomach acid, to the absorption of nutrients, to the elimination of waste. Eating at the same time of day, every day, helps to normalize these processes.

The synchronization with our master clock, set by light exposure, played a critical role in helping our ancestral bodies regulate themselves over the seasons. As the light signal diminished in strength, at temperate latitudes, at least, moving from summer to fall, and eventually into the depths of winter, the length of time our digestive system would be "on" gradually decreased. This makes a lot of sense given that food was less abundant during the winter months relative to spring and summer. There's no point in having a system hungry and ready to consume if no appreciable amount of food is forthcoming. Not to mention that the digestive system requires energy and other resources to function (think of all the enzymes, hormones, bile, acid, and so on it produces).

Our digestive physiology, like many other systems in our body, is linked to the light, and is seemingly at its most efficient when we eat most of our food early in the day, and wind down our energy intake toward the early evening. In sum, the research in this area confirms the old adage of eating breakfast like a king, lunch like a prince, and dinner like a pauper.

As the light intensity and day length ebbs and flows across the year with the changing seasons, so, too, does the feeding window over which it is best for us to eat: longer in summer, shorter in winter. Factor in what should be the natural variations in food availability over the seasons, and you have the makings of a dietary pattern that keeps everyone happy. You have periods of high vegetable and fruit consumption, periods of lower-carbohydrate, higher-fat consumption, periods of extended fasting, a bigger variation in protein sources across the course of a year, and eating patterns matched to our ever-shifting circadian rhythms. In other words, our ancestors did practice intermittent fasting—they just did so in winter. They ate low carb—sometimes. They were "plant-based"—sometimes.

Rhythmicity in eating might all sound good in theory, but it doesn't fit neatly into how we behave in modern society. Our pattern of continuous energy consumption over so many hours is exactly the strategy many animals deploy in the height of summer and into fall in order to increase their body fat levels for the next winter. As a child, I saw this in the black bears that often showed up on my parents' property to forage for everything and anything to eat as they sensed the cold winter approaching. This problem is compounded by the fact that most modern people, most of the time, consume most of their energy from main meals (both protein and nonprotein) in the evening, often well after sunset, leading to a mismatch in circadian rhythm signals. If that isn't bad enough, recall that many people spend their days in relatively low light conditions ("winter light"). Talk about confusing your body with inconsistent—or incoherent—messages!

People keep chronic summer hours, spend time in chronic winter light, and get chronic summer sleep, all while chronically consuming a summer dieting schedule—all irrespective of what the actual season happens to be. From a circadian biology standpoint alone, this is a perfect recipe for metabolic disorders and other adverse health consequences. I don't believe that most people consciously choose this lifestyle. They simply participate in the environment that has been built around them. They must go to work early and often return home late. They don't control their daytime light exposure, and didn't curate the menu of cheap, hyperpalatable carbohydrate-dense food that surrounds them. It isn't easy to opt out of all of this, even when we're well educated and well resourced, but it's possible. Many dietary strategies see people concerned about eating locally, reducing food waste and packaging, and ensuring that the foods they source are raised and grown as healthfully, ethically, and sustainably as possible. These are laudable goals, and they are important. Now we just need to add seasonal rhythms and circadian biology to the mix. Don't worry, this all comes together with a lot more ease than you might think.

Make It a Family Affair

Even if we pay attention to what and when we are eating (no small feat!), we often neglect one of the most important aspects of our modern food and nutrition landscape: whom we are chowing down with. Go to Europe, South America, or Asia, and you'll notice a striking difference in food consumption. In these regions, broadly speaking, people rarely eat on the move, and they eat alone a lot less often than in North America. You'll be hard-pressed to find anyone walking down the street with a burger in one hand and a soda in the other. Meals are generally sit-down affairs, enjoyed in the company of others.

Social engagement is a hallmark of the most long-lived communities and societies around the world—the so-called Blue Zones.[17] One important aspect of this social engagement is the coming together to prepare and share meals, to break bread together, as it were. Social eating is a timeless human ritual with deep evolutionary roots. Research suggests that people who eat more socially tend to be happier and more satisfied, trust others more, and interact more in their own communities.[18] They even have a larger support system. Recent research shows that eating *the same food* with others increases the sense of trust and cooperation.[19] Food literally brings us closer to friends and strangers alike.

Eating together might have evolved as a way for us to connect and bond socially. And yet, Americans rarely eat together anymore. Food journalist Michael Pollan estimates that Americans consume at least one in every five meals in their cars.[20] Almost 40 percent (36.6) of Americans eat at least one fast-food meal every single day—ultra-processed foods specifically designed to be eaten with one hand, on the go.[21] As I've observed in my consultant practice, many American families don't prioritize sharing meals together at all, and often only eat together a couple of times a week.[22] Even when families, couples, and friends do eat together, it is often in a state of distraction, in front of the television, or worse, with smartphones and video games present. More people are also eating alone, compounding any feelings of isolation and loneliness they already experience. I'm always saddened when

I witness a food hall full of individuals eating alone, often soothing their loneliness, or at least distracting themselves from it, by scrolling their phones or computers between bites.

In the more socialized countries of Europe and the Mediterranean region, the midday meal is often the day's most important, with workers taking long lunch breaks. In such countries, it is often culturally frowned upon to eat in a rush and while on the go. The French, for instance, tend to eat together as a household more regularly and to follow a regular pattern of three meals a day.

In North America, Britain, and Australia, where society is more individualistic and convenience often dictates food choices, you see a greater consumption of energy-dense, highly processed fast foods and snacks. You also see a more entrenched culture of meal skipping. Yet the health authorities of these very same countries revere the Mediterranean diet as the model for how we all should eat. In so doing, they homogenize and distill the distinct and varied diets of the Mediterranean region to a few pithy, sound bite–like recommendations (eat fish and olive oil, they say, or nuts, or certain spices) without ever properly addressing the wider culture and context of eating in these regions. Mediterranean peoples eat simply, regularly, together, in a state of relaxation, without digital distraction, and largely without deliberate restriction. That's a diet I can wholeheartedly endorse.

Accessing Our Intuition

As I've been arguing, we must all develop a more holistic approach to eating, starting with the food we select. If we find ourselves in the throes of chronic summer and are habituated to highly rewarding flavors and tastes, healthy or whole foods will have zero appeal. Before we can gain any awareness of our deep, intuitive yearning for seasonally appropriate, nutritious food, we must first extricate ourselves from the overstimulation of summer foods. If we're used to nutrient-poor inflammatory foods, like Cheetos and Diet Coke—or even "healthy" summer foods like processed granola bars and white rice—we'll never be drawn to salmon and summer squash.

Here's a simple rubric: limit your diet to the food available at your local farmers' market. Ask local farmers the most important questions about your diet: What are you making right now? What are you growing? What are you producing? If you adopt this practice of food selection, you'll be about 75 percent of the way into seasonal eating. But be cautious. I've begun to see farmers' market vendors offer foods from global suppliers and grocery stores, like strawberries in November or winter squashes in the spring. If you spot such offerings at your local market, steer clear, and make sure you only select *locally* grown and produced food. You might also consult my book *It Starts with Food*. My coauthor and I outline a diet that represents a moderate midpoint between the seasonal extremes of summer and winter. It helps readers move beyond a modern, refined agricultural diet based on grains and legumes to better food choices.

Once you're selecting foods properly, you can begin to tap into your intuition about eating. When I first started paying attention to seasonality and food, I quickly noticed that I wasn't interested in eating fruit during the winter months. It was during the cold and dark month of January, and I was living in Maine. I'm not a picky eater, and I broadly gravitate to fruits and vegetables of all kinds. But I just didn't *feel like* eating any fruit. This wasn't based on any preconceived diet or idea about what I *should* eat. It was an intuition about what was good and nourishing for my body in that context.

Once you start eating seasonal offerings at your farmers' markets or have completed a round of the Whole30 diet, you'll start to discover such intuitions. New personal wisdom about your body will emerge. But it takes time to distinguish cravings from intuitive longings for seasonally appropriate foods. Have you ever noticed that when you experience a craving, you gravitate toward sweet, salty, and fatty foods, and that it comes on pretty strong? Sugar supplies a calorie-dense and almost immediately available energy source, while salt helps us balance our electrolytes. Animal protein sources represent the most energy-dense food, which is why every now and then you might have a hankering for a thick piece of marbled steak or short ribs. Unfortunately, processed foods have allowed us to satisfy our cravings with place-holder foods and chemical triggers—chips, cookies, MSG (which provides *umami*—that savory, meaty taste), and the like—that don't nourish or satiate us. If you work hard to overcome the appeal of these fake foods, you might just wake up one spring morning and say to yourself, "For some reason, a fresh green salad with strawberries and marcona almonds sounds delicious today."

I hope I've persuaded you that what we eat should fluctuate with the seasons. But how about our movement patterns? Here, the science isn't as straightforward. Still, just as with food, we need to develop our intuitive capacities to switch from chronic summer movement patterns to simpler fall and winter modes. A substantial portion of the population is either stuck on chronic summer workout patterns or is completely sedentary. But as we'll explore next, these consistent modes of exercise, or lack thereof, have compromised our bodily integrity, our health, and our longevity. In order to be fully functional and flourishing human beings, we must restore the ancestral fluctuations in our movement patterns. Too bad there's no "farmers' market rule" for movement!

CHAPTER FOUR

Moving to the Rhythm

James was tired of *working for the man* in the daily nine-to-five office grind. He woke up early to catch the subway into the office and ended his days in much the same way. He could only make it to the gym after work, and while it made for a long day, it provided him a sorely needed stress release after being chained to a desk. James chafed under this weekly routine and dreamed of working for himself, building a robust online platform, and then cracking the big time as a social media influencer. As a self-employed entrepreneur, instead of a corporate shill, he figured he'd have more autonomy and flexibility—the freedom to do what he wanted, when he wanted, including hitting the gym whenever he liked and traveling to exotic places like all the "influencers" seemed to be doing all the time.

James eventually quit his job and began working for himself at home. He soon discovered that producing high-quality content for his channels and staying ahead of his competition wasn't easy. To keep pace, he changed his routine dramatically. In order to post initial content before viewers scrolled their social media feeds at breakfast or on their daily commutes, James began getting up earlier in the morning. He also stayed up later and later so as to keep up on all the social interactions on his channels. In order to maximize those all-important likes and subscribes, he had to pay constant round-the-clock attention to his screens, leaving him only a few bleary hours of shut-eye every night.

After a few months of this new schedule, James saw a marked deterioration in his physical fitness and an increase in his body fat levels. As he realized, he had replaced a nine-to-five with a five-to-nine (if not worse), and was no longer walking twice a day to and from the subway. He seldom made it to the gym and was less focused when he did go, posting Instagram stories along the way. James had swapped *working for the man* with *working for a computer algorithm,* endlessly chasing hits, likes, subscribers, and comments. The algorithm was proving to be a much more demanding boss, and James was paying the price.

James's story points us to a sad truth about technology. We now have labor-saving devices like computers in every home, constant connectivity throughout the world, and the ability to work from anywhere, largely according to our own schedules. But do we have more free time for physical activity as a result? Not at all. Instead, the industrial, technological, information, and social media revolutions have eroded the boundaries and blurred the lines between our professional and private lives, between home and away. Thanks to the powerful computer in our pockets, we are constantly connected to the office, and moving less than ever before, regardless of our occupation or industry.

We also increasingly spend what leisure time we do have in front of screens. American adults spend almost 50 percent of their days, or more than ten hours, with their noses buried in their tablets, smartphones, computers, and televisions.[1] In 2016, American adults also logged nearly six and a half hours of sitting a day, probably looking at screens.[2] Such sitting time is harmful—to quote a CNN headline, reporting on a 2017 *Annals of Internal Medicine* study, "Yes, sitting too long can kill you, even if you exercise."[3] Unfortunately, most adults don't exercise either. As a 2018 World Health Organization (WHO) study found, only 25 percent of global adults engage in enough physical activity, which per the study left "more than 1.4 billion adults at risk of developing or exacerbating diseases linked to inactivity."[4]

The situation is even bleaker for younger Americans. Of the five and a half hours of free time that American teens have each day, the Pew Research Center found they spent the majority (almost three hours on weekdays and nearly four hours on weekends) scrolling, swiping, surfing, and playing games on screens.[5] Year after year, in tests assessing physical fitness and strength, children have become weaker and less aerobically fit. "Kids today are less fit than their parents were," proclaimed the *Washington Post* in 2013, echoing many such headlines since. Citing a series of studies analyzing millions of children throughout the world, the article demonstrated that today's kids had fitness levels significantly inferior to those of their parents.[6] This was true across different genders and ages, and probably struck most as unsurprising. Schools have scaled back physical education programs, and participation in organized sports hasn't generally increased over the years.[7] Parents and educators tend to believe that maintaining optimal physical fitness, and understanding how one's body works, isn't as important for the future as, say, learning how to code or score high on a college entrance test. And this pervasive attitude directly harms our youth. According to Sam Kass, a former White House chef and head of Michelle Obama's Let's Move initiative, "We are currently facing the most sedentary generation of children in our history."[8]

Everything from the removal of sidewalks (often to widen roads and allow better traffic flow), to fears for children's safety, to increasing traffic on school routes has resulted in children walking and cycling less and being driven to school and extracurricular activities. Notice the irony. Anxious parents drive their tired and unfit children to school, increasing the traffic and pollution around schools while reinforcing their fears about the dangers of walking or biking. This in turn further deteriorates our kids' physical fitness levels. It's a vicious, sedentary cycle.

Previous generations of children and adolescents may have sought to get out of the house to hang out, *in person*, with their friends. For today's kids, access to Wi-Fi is paramount, and with more and more children having their own smartphone at a young age, the constant connection these devices afford means kids are even less likely to leave home and move. According to the WHO, only 20 percent of global youth get enough exercise.[9] In 2019, the WHO publicized new guidelines suggesting that "to grow up healthy, children need to sit less and play more."[10]

All of us have to get ourselves moving—but how exactly? As I'll discuss more later in the book, we must first establish a baseline pattern of movement in our lives—an "anchor," as I call it—by reintroducing activities like easy walking, hiking, taking the stairs, and electing to carry our personal items. Once we recover a measure of the physical strength that our ancestors likely enjoyed, we can go on to optimize our health and longevity by slightly modifying our movements on a seasonal basis. As we'll find, our renewed dedication to physical strength will increase our longevity and quality of life, leaving us with strong, resilient, and happy bodies over a long life span.

"Working Out," Caveman Style

Did our distant ancestors really work out? Of course not. They didn't need to, because in the course of their daily lives they engaged in a broad range of physical activities, like walking, carrying, lifting, and the occasional sprint to flee from a hostile predator or violent adversary. Based on what we know about our ancestors' lifestyles, we might characterize their fundamental and basic movements as including the following three elements:

- They undertook a relatively high volume of lower-intensity, high-frequency activities such as walking, with much of it performed as incidental physical activity throughout the day. They simply moved.
- They loaded their muscles, bones, and connective tissues by engaging in lifting and carrying movements, beginning with body weight and progressively increasing the loads over time. They lifted and carried heavy things.
- They undertook a relatively low volume of high-intensity activity, such as sprinting, doing so after building a strong foundation with both lower-intensity and higher-loading (lifting and carrying) activities. They ran like hell occasionally.

Early on in my thinking, I transposed this three-part movement oscillation onto my seasonal model, arriving at broad generalizations about how our preindustrial human ancestors moved. Summer, with its longer days and warmer temperatures, lent itself to doing more work—gathering, hunting, child rearing, and resource exploration—all in preparation for the coming winter. The amount of activity was high, but its intensity remained low. Come winter, at least at high latitudes, the amount of activity decreased. It would have been too brutally cold to stay outside for very long, and the daylight hours too short to venture on long explorations. But with a need to gather food (predominantly from hunting), retrieve water (possibly frozen), and lug wood for the fire, the overall relative intensity of winter activity would still have been considerable.

While this is a convenient shorthand for my model, I now realize that life for our ancestors wasn't this consistent or straightforward. Not every tribal society would have remained in one place across the year. Many tribes would have migrated, keeping pace with roaming herds and flocks, or ventured to more hospitable climes during winter. Many ancestral societies would see a mixture of the three main elements I've outlined: a lot of relatively low-intensity movement and a lot of lifting and carrying, punctuated by infrequent and intermittent bursts of high-intensity activity (once again: think running from a hostile lion). While the relative balance of these elements might have changed seasonally to a certain extent, I don't believe the pendulum would have swung all that far. Indeed, of all my four keys, I now feel that movement and physical activity are perhaps the *least* oscillatory, relative to sleep, diet, and even social connection.

I'm not saying that varying our movement patterns is unimportant. Think of food. While we lack details about Paleo man and woman's caloric expenditures and exercise routines, we do know that they were incredibly resilient, adaptable, and varied in their diets and movements—they were food and movement omnivores, so to speak. Humans are incredibly adaptable. For the sake of our health and well-being, we should strive to be so, too, engaging in nourishing movements like lifting and carrying that bolster our musculoskeletal and nervous systems, rendering us capable and durable. Ancestral movement patterns functioned atop a physical foundation of strength (lifting and carrying), with most movement occurring at a relatively low intensity (walking) but punctuated by relatively short bouts of high-intensity movement (sprinting). The totality of these ancestral movements resulted in what physical therapists and fitness practitioners now call excellent general physical preparation (GPP).

Within this general rootedness in broad-based movement, our ancestors likely varied their physical activities to some degree. Consider the evolutionary imperative of high-intensity physical activity. Our ancestors would have needed and utilized short bursts of speed and power in a variety of scenarios, ranging from the final lunge to make a kill to the fight-or-flight response from predators (including other humans). In our ancestral environments, you couldn't out-jog tigers or flash floods. Short-burst activities would have oscillated on a semi-seasonal basis (think of hunting season versus migration season), strengthening our ancestors' bodies and increasing their survival rates and vitality. They would have also improved certain metabolic pathways, making our ancestors better at converting carbohydrates into cellular energy, and helping them control and clear lactic acid from their muscles. When performing low-intensity, general physical activity, like migrating when the weather was bad or when following a herd of animals, our ancestors would have enhanced more metabolic pathways, making their bodies more effective at using fat as a fuel source. Ultimately, their varied movements would have increased the range of their bodies' capacities, enabling them to not just survive but thrive in different environments and under different conditions.

We moderns should return to such oscillatory movements to enhance different metabolic pathways and render our bodies stronger and more resilient. Such movement oscillation, however, looks different than it did with nutrition. When I described the seasonal oscillation model with nutrition in chapter 3, you may have visualized a circle with four quadrants, each representing the four seasons. When it comes to movement, visualize instead an elongated ellipse. Spring and summer run along one edge of the ellipse and fall and winter along the other. With this visual in mind, you can think of roughly varying your workouts not among the four seasons, but rather between two general poles of winter and summer. In performing these two major oscillations, you're providing your body the opportunity to adapt to different stimuli, which serve to strengthen our bodies, just like it did our ancestors'.

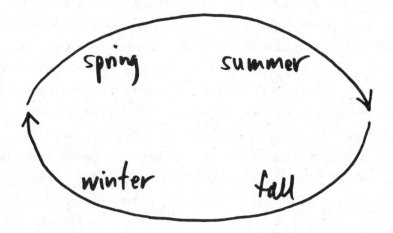

With movement, as with nutrition, the summer/fall and winter/spring transitions matter most. The transition from winter to spring is relatively easy to accomplish because, as dopamine-driven, novelty-seeking human beings, we spontaneously seek expansion in the springtime, getting into the garden, doing spring-cleaning, and starting a new exercise program. In the summer months, generally speaking, we should incorporate large volumes and long durations of general movement, like hiking and being out and about at the park or the lake. Think of the classic summertime staples of bike rides and throwing the

Frisbee for your dog or with your kids. As we enjoy mostly pleasant weather outside, we should choose to do a lot more walking and carrying, like rambling to the grocery store and ferrying our groceries back home. Here you might pause and think, "I'll look crazy if I walk a mile to the store!" Yes, you might, by conventional standards. In modern society, most people don't leave the car at home and deliberately move their bodies instead. But we must substitute convenience for movement, because our society's default is movement minimization. And if the headlines are right, we'll soon miss even the short walk to our cars as we head to the supermarket, since most of our groceries will arrive at home via drone delivery. Have you seen the animated film *Wall-E?* Yeah, it'll be like that.

The winter-to-spring shift might be easy, but the difficult transition—and the place where we can easily become stuck—is the pivot from summer to fall. We've observed how the last ten thousand years of human history, premised on agriculture and civilization, orients us to the logic of summer—the allure of expansion, craving, dopamine, pleasure, ease. Whether it's staying up late, feasting on carbohydrate-rich foods, or basking in artificial light, it's easy to get stuck in summer. The same holds true for movement. As the leaves change color and the colder weather approaches, we'll naturally begin spending less time outdoors, and thus doing less general movement. Our whole world, literally and figuratively, should contract during these months as we spend more time resting and nesting at home.

But just because we experience an overall reduction in the duration of our activities doesn't mean we should become sedentary in these months. Instead, we should vary our movements, substituting longer, easier workouts with shorter, harder, interval-based or sprint-based training. We should also adjust the nature of physical connections. Summertime lends itself to outdoor activities with lots of people—we enjoy the excitement of exploring groups and the rush of meeting new acquaintances. Running a 10K with a bunch of friends makes good summertime sense. In the fall and winter, the nature of our movements changes, as our more indoor and concentrated efforts, performed among close family and friends, entail more intimacy and vulnerability. Think of working with a personal coach, or training with a gym buddy.

Our movement patterns should thus obey the oscillatory logic we've seen throughout this book. Fall's and spring's movement should be moderate in both intensity and duration, but only as transition points between the more polarized movement extremes of summer and winter. The pivot from summer to fall—and from winter to spring—represents a moderation of both intensity and duration, where winter itself sees more of a reduction in total activity by duration and time, and an introduction to short, hard, interval-based or sprint-based training that isn't present at all in the summertime.

Let's say you wanted to take up a competitive sport like running, and to oscillate your training seasonally. In the spring, you might begin by engaging in low-intensity, moderate-duration preparation. You're just getting started. This would represent your aerobic period early in the training season and should be full of low-intensity runs, or something referred to in the lingo as "base building." As you get more fit, you can lengthen your training sessions. As you approached the date of your event, be it a ten-kilometer run, half marathon, or ultra-marathon, summer's long training would gradually yield to fall, and you would reduce your overall exercise duration. At this juncture, you would increase your overall intensity, training closer to your aerobic thresholds, or doing some sprint work and "sharpening" activities. But you would also want to scale back or eliminate your long, base-building runs in turn. This transition from summer to fall wouldn't be stark, nor look significantly different. It would simply involve a tapering off general activity, and a ramping up of intensity. Picture a sine wave, not a right angle.

Unfortunately, whether we're preparing for a race or simply going about our days, we don't tend to maintain a foundation of basic daily movement, accompanied by slight seasonal oscillations. Most of us are slaves to our environments, which naturally lead us to move very little. While my writing here is a nudge (if not a vigorous shove) in the direction of a high degree of "healthy deviancy" from the status quo (to use the term coined by my dear friend Pilar Gerasimo), we can only opt out of our environment so much without becoming misfits or outcasts or risk losing the jobs we depend on. If you work away from home for ten or twelve hours every day, you probably won't break out the vacuum cleaner each night just to elevate your heart rate. If you live on the seventh floor of an apartment building, I don't expect you will volunteer to carry buckets of water up and down the stairs for an hour, as great as this may be as a workout. Without being too extreme, or arousing the concern of our neighbors, we must find ways to reintroduce a basic level of movement into our lives. Then, and only then, can we begin to oscillate those movements on a seasonal basis.

Become an Exercise Generalist

So, what should we do—get on that treadmill more often? Hop on a stationary bike or attend CrossFit classes three times a week? It's not so simple—these and other popular forms of exercise are actually part of the problem. Ours is a world where you can shop online for a robotic vacuum cleaner so that you no longer need to vacuum your home (because who has time for that?), while at the same time you must buy exercise equipment or a gym membership to ride a stationary bike or walk on a treadmill to improve your cardiovascular health. Just like the standard American diet has stripped the nourishing components out of naturally occurring nutrient-dense foods and replaced them with ultra-processed, nutrient-poor food products, so we've stripped the nourishing movements from our everyday life. In the name of efficiency, productivity, and ease, we've stopped walking, carrying, pushing, and lifting—the very activities that make us strong, functional, and durable humans for decades. Then we reincorporate some form of (processed) movement back into our lives via our regular exercise programs.

As the brilliant biomechanist Katy Bowman has observed, humans have transitioned from movement generalists to movement specialists. We now perform an ever-narrowing range of movements that leave us overtaxed in some areas and undernourished in others.[11] Think of factory workers performing the same repetitive tasks hundreds or thousands of times per day. (As a physical therapist, I often treated "overuse" and "repetitive strain" injuries.) Or office workers whose movement specialization entails being seated at a desk and pecking away at a keyboard, gaze fixed on their screen. Many of us, regardless of occupation, outsource our baseline needs, like acquiring food, shelter, and fuel, to the specialized movements of others, and then only engage in highly specialized movements as it relates to a singular sport or exercise, such as running, cycling, or tennis. When it comes to movement, we're effectively eating potato chips and chocolate bars, and then consuming a multivitamin (i.e., a narrowly defined, non-oscillatory activity), and expecting to be healthy.

It's true that in order to fulfill a large chunk of the three major elements of movement I outlined above, most modern humans must engage in some form of planned and structured physical activity, exercise, and training. And many people choose to do just that. But the classic mistake is to go from low levels of any activity to immediately specializing in one, like jogging, cycling, or obstacle-course racing, and performing said activity at virtually the same frequency, intensity, and time (duration) all year-round. Consider the jogger who shuffles around the park at the same speed every day, for years on end, not getting any fitter or faster, but nursing a progressively deteriorating lower back, hips, and knees. The frequency is the same. The intensity is the same. The duration is the same. There is no oscillation. Things get worse over time.

Those starting out with high-intensity interval training programs, such as CrossFit, often fare similarly. They begin well enough with high-intensity, relatively short-duration (e.g., ten minutes), low-frequency (e.g., one to two days per week) workouts, all of which contain some variation (read: oscillation). But then, slowly, people's participation tends to increase to year-round high-intensity workouts, with increased duration (either longer classes or multiple classes per day), higher frequency (five to six days per week), and no real oscillation. These athletes become increasingly exhausted and their relative effort in each workout slumps. Soon enough, the six-days-a-week, twenty-minute CrossFitter is flatlining on the same "chronic cardio" as the six-days-a-week, twenty-minute park jogger. Doing different movements but using the same metabolic pathways isn't true variation.

I often see destructive chronic cardio patterns among weekend warriors—people who engage in demanding physical activity during their off-time, which usually falls on the weekend. Many of them choose activities that afford little to no oscillation in their movements. They live a largely sedentary life during the week, not engaging in general activities like walking, lifting, carrying, or real-life functional strength movements. On weekends, during mountain biking workouts or recreation league soccer games, they push their bodies really hard. Such weekend warriors oscillate, but in a destructive way: they work too hard on their chosen specialties when they should be taking it easy, and take it too easy (perhaps because they are too tired and worn out from previous workouts) when they should be pushing a bit harder. They aggregate toward a middle ground, maintained across the year, that is both too stressful at moments and not stressful enough at other times to develop a healthy baseline of fitness and physical conditioning.

One need only glimpse nonindustrialized traditional cultures to see evidence of our generalist roots. In such cultures, people still use basic, labor-intensive tools, replicating the broad movement patterns that drove the evolution of our physical attributes and capacities. In contrast to modern, industrialized, automobile-centric societies, members of traditional cultures walk. A lot. In fact, they engage in a relatively high volume of light-to-moderate walking, in the range of three to ten miles per day. With the exception of those engaging in some form of intentional cardiovascular exercise, most people in modern society cover less than three miles per day at a comparable intensity. Yes, even those with a Fitbit who walk around the block during their lunch breaks (which I do encourage!).

Members of nonindustrialized and traditional cultures move their bodies at a relatively low-to-moderate level of intensity across a wide range of activities. Those whom modern societies deem "fit" or "active," by contrast, often participate in specialized sports or exercise, instead of more general activity. Modern people accumulate this activity at much higher relative intensities and sustain that intensity for much longer periods of time. Imagine covering ten miles across a day through such acts as fetching water, sourcing and preparing food, firewood, and other supplies, undertaking general chores, and maybe engaging in social activities or dance. Compare this to a typically modern scenario of driving everywhere, remaining seated most of the day, and then going for a six-to-ten-mile run at 80 percent of your maximum heart rate a few times a week. The former group is likely aerobically fit and strong, yet we wouldn't think of them as such because they are not, in our modern eyes, performing a distinct, specialized fitness session.

Also consider the surface areas on which these activities unfold. In traditional societies, people living in major towns and villages walk or run on dirt, sand, and rough ground. This aids in the development of foot and hip strength and stability, promoting balance and protecting the body from falls and strains. Most modern cities feature flat, uniform surfaces of asphalt and concrete. As the *Guardian* evocatively put it, "Concrete is modernity's foundation stone: it surrounds us in bridges, motorways, tunnels, hospitals, stadiums and churches—from the Roman Pantheon, which is what God might pour if he had a concrete mixer, to Clifton Cathedral in Bristol, which looks like the ashtray where he would stub out his cigarettes."[12]

These compact surfaces might accommodate the modern corporate uniform of heavy, tight-fitting clothing and restrictive, heeled shoes, but walking, jogging, and running on them for even moderate distances can promote repetitive strain-type injuries to bone and connective tissue. And you don't even have to run. Teachers, nurses, engineers, and others who spend a lot of time merely standing on hard floors can experience a painful foot-based inflammation called plantar fasciitis, as well as osteoarthritis, Achilles tendonitis, and even varicose veins.[13] Of course, we typically address these maladies with more cushioning, controlling footwear, and anti-inflammatory steroid injections—strategies that often cause more problems than they fix.

Perhaps of greater significance to our current well-being is not *cardiovascular* activity, as we in the modern world call it, but activities of daily living that strengthen our *musculoskeletal system*, such as lifting, carrying, climbing, and throwing. People undertake such activities from a very early age in traditional egalitarian societies, continuing throughout their lives. If you have ever watched *National Geographic*–type documentaries on such societies, you would have seen the classic images of a woman carrying baskets of food, bundles of firewood, or large bunches of bananas on her head, often with a child wrapped around her hip. You might have watched this from the comfort of your couch and thought, "Poor woman!" Such high musculoskeletal-load activities, however, allow for the development of physical strength not seen in most modern, urbanized humans. That "poor woman" might face many issues in her life, but those don't include a frail and weak body. She'll be strong and independent for the duration of her life. Compare that to the ten million Americans who have osteoporosis and the forty-four million more who suffer from poor bone density.[14]

In their paper "Achieving Hunter-Gatherer Fitness in the 21(st) Century," James O'Keefe and his coauthors produced a table of typical hunter-gatherer activities and their modern-day equivalents.[15] Our ancestors performed high-load activities like carrying baskets of gathered food or wood while we moderns carry bags of groceries or luggage. It might sound equivalent, but it's not. Our modern penchant for labor-saving conveniences has worked against us in each of these cases. Carrying our belongings has now become dragging luggage on low-friction wheels. Carrying children has become pushing them in strollers. Small, low-maintenance yards have rendered our gardening activities less extensive and strenuous. Wood, if you even need it, might come to your door presplit, and if you pay enough, they might even stack it for you.

The removal of these "burdens," no matter how welcome we might find it, leads our muscles and bones to weaken from disuse. We then break them down even further via inflammatory diets, stress, lack of sleep, and insufficient sunlight exposure. These effects have their own scientific names: *dynapenia* (loss of muscular power), *sarcopenia* (loss of muscle mass), and *osteopenia* (loss of bone density). All three form an often silent, interrelated triad of decreasing physical health and function. These *pervasive penias* (as I have heard one exercise physiologist call them) grow increasingly apparent earlier in our life spans than we've ever seen historically. In traditional societies, elderly people often perform hard physical labor well into their sixties, seventies, and eighties. What strikes us as unusual and awkward activities—like carrying water on our heads or squatting for extended lengths of time—keeps people strong and functional over their lifetimes.

The effects of reduced muscular load in modern life are similar to what astronauts experience after spending prolonged periods of time in a zero-gravity environment. When we rely on a chair to support our bodies instead of our bones, muscles, and connective tissues, we are effectively creating a low-gravity environment. Something similar holds true when we use carts, elevators, and cars to move objects. It might take years of exposure to such low-effort conditions here on earth to match the deterioration experienced over only a few weeks and months by astronauts in space. But such physical deterioration undoubtedly takes its toll. We tend to shrug it off as "getting old," but it's not—it's the product of unhealthy aging, driven by years and years of mistreating our bodies.

Bear in mind that our muscles aren't just the mechanisms that move us. They also function as a secretory organ, and they release chemical messengers into the body, like your pancreas or thyroid gland. These messengers, called myokines, help to control your metabolism, as well as bone and immune health. Myokines also help to protect us from excessive inflammation (driven by inflammatory cytokines), and are present in proportion to our movement and muscle mass.[16] I'm always frustrated by the commonly distorted meme suggesting that "you can't outrun a poor diet." It became popular in the mid-2000s to underscore the importance of good nutrition *and* physical fitness, not one or the other.[17] I find that the adage mainly reinforces the notion that you really only need to follow a particular type of diet such as low carb or keto, and that strenuous muscular contraction doesn't matter very much. That's a dangerous, misleading conclusion.

While physical activity guidelines have recommended some form of weight-bearing or muscle-building exercise for decades, such prescriptions remain vague, if not outright glib. The US Department of Health and Human Services began releasing guidelines to help inform Americans about the importance of physical movement and health beginning in 2008.[18] Some of their key findings include, "Adults should move more and sit less throughout the day" and "some physical activity is better than none."[19] They also recommend several key staples of good fitness, including moderate-to-vigorous cardiovascular/aerobic exercise, stretching and flexibility exercises, and even the development and maintenance of total body strength across a life span (though the overall emphasis still seems to be on cardiovascular health).

According to Todd Miller, an associate professor in the Department of Exercise Science at George Washington University, everyone should engage in strength training, but only about one in five Americans follow government exercise guidelines.[20] But even for the 20 percent of Americans who do, these guidelines remain a starting point at best. Taking them at face value, it's hard to know how to build muscle and bone strength safely and effectively to achieve a good range of movement through the joints (and people actually need range of motion more than the muscular flexibility they chase through stretching). Even more important, how do we actually develop the cardiovascular system? For all the emphasis on "heart health" and cardiovascular disease prevention, we shouldn't forget: the heart is a muscle too.

The average person will probably associate strength training with bodybuilding, big muscles, and testosterone-filled gymnasiums full of grunting men. This perception, married to the public health and media bias toward cardio-based exercise, and the common understanding that weight loss requires us to "burn calories," accounts for the popular notion that cardio is "king." People think that the best way to burn a lot of calories is to perform exercises that lead to an increased and sustained heart rate. Gyms, moreover, are expensive and difficult to get to. It's much easier to slap on a pair of running shoes or hop on a stationary bike and get your heart rate up.

In truth, poor cardiovascular fitness isn't what stops you from picking up your three-year-old grandchild or getting out of a chair in your eighties. An efficient heart isn't what stops you from falling over and breaking a bone should you lose balance. You interact with the world either by exerting force against something (for instance, walking up a flight of stairs) or by resisting the forces being applied to your body and dissipating their effect (for instance, minimizing the impact of a fall). For all of us, and especially women, gaining more physical strength allows us to engage more fully and self-confidently with the world than virtually any other exercise modality, and this is especially true as we age.

In recent years, high-intensity interval training has been the exercise modality *du jour*. HIIT programs might feature single bouts of maximum-effort sprints, or the classic (though potentially overused) Tabata intervals of twenty-second efforts interspersed with ten-second rest intervals and repeated eight times.[21] Rooted in the circuit training of yesteryear, HIIT represents a welcome departure from traditional physical activity guidelines that have focused on high-frequency exercise most days of the week, at a moderate to vigorous intensity, and at relatively longer durations. Over the last couple of decades, more research has focused on the benefits of lower-frequency and higher-intensity training. Working through slightly different physiological pathways than the classic continuous aerobic exercise, these high-intensity intervals have proven themselves to be as beneficial as high-frequency, lower-intensity, longer-duration exercise, if not more. They've been shown to enhance overall fitness and wellness levels, not to mention decrease blood pressure and help control blood sugar levels.[22]

Exerting yourself at near maximum effort is structurally hard on the body, though, especially tendons, joints, and ligaments. We condition such tissues by undertaking a great deal of low-intensity movement each day, as our ancestors did via the many different types of lifting and carrying they performed. Once we restore our baseline physical fitness levels, we'll be ready for such activity too. That's because we're almost hardwired to move in the right ways. Children tend to be natural sprinters, engaging in relatively short bursts of effort interspersed with longer periods of lower-intensity movement. Older readers may still remember how children used to develop strong physical conditioning via rough-and-tumble natural play, spontaneous dancing or wrestling, school physical education programs based on gymnastics or calisthenics, or the trialing of several sports.

Funding cuts for school physical education programs, greater emphasis on academics and technological savvy over physical health and development, the sad state of health care, technology additions, and a host of other factors have all made children less inclined to stay active. When children do select some form of physical activity, they often opt for a relatively specialized and highly repetitive sport. These weak, unfit children, who may have had quite negative experiences with physical activity, grow into weak, unfit adults who fail to prioritize physical capacity. Carry this effect across a couple of generations, and being relatively weak and unfit becomes the new normal.

Overcoming Polarization

Our extremes of excessively consistent, monotonous movement or a lack of exertion altogether form what we might term a *polarization* in movement. What we truly need is more of a balance or middle ground. Research examining the training of elite athletes suggests that most of their training (upward of 80 percent) takes place at relatively low to moderate intensities, while specific workouts relevant to their sport, state, and stage of competitive season take place at relatively high intensities.[23] That is, they spend little time occupying the two polar extremes. Far from a concept applicable exclusively to elite athletes, this is a useful way for us everyday athletes to organize our own physical activity.

Starting out, you might want to perform low-intensity movements by taking a brisk walk or going for a leisurely swim or bike ride. At least 80 to 90 percent of your exercise volume should focus in this zone. This kind of movement shouldn't feel very stressful, and should include other aspects of health such as natural light, time outside, interpersonal connection, and avoidance of smartphones and other screens. At the opposite extreme of the intensity scale, you should perform a few short sprints at the highest relative intensity you can manage. In practice, we might be talking about three hours of walking per week plus two ten-minute sessions of sprint-like movement, where each sprint-like effort might last five to thirty seconds.

Sandwiched between these two polarized extremes, forming the critical foundation for most people's structured exercise routines, should be some form of progressive strength training. Given that we can't necessarily change our environments to allow for more strength-building loads on our bones and muscles, working deliberately to make our bodies stronger is one of the most essential things we can do for our health. Strength training programs can range from body-weight movements (such as calisthenics or yoga), to using tools like dumbbells and kettlebells, to specific barbell and powerlifting programs. Yes, walking and sprinting are good, but neither will benefit you as much if you lack underlying musculoskeletal strength. Build strength first, develop cardio second.

In line with my seasonal model, we should oscillate these activities over the year. The long daylight hours and hotter temperatures of summer lend themselves to longer, lower-intensity physical efforts. Shorter, colder winter days lend themselves to emphasize high-intensity efforts, with perhaps the occasional longer, lower-intensity effort if the weather allows. Year-round, continue building foundational, core strength by engaging in lifting, carrying, and smaller, easier shifts like taking the stairs. Also, don't forget to share these activities with others. The rush of sharing a thrilling descent on a mountain bike with a friend will bond you together. I'm not suggesting that authentic human connection can only happen in physical environments and circumstances. But, in my experience, the bonds formed hiking up a mountain versus driving to the same point are much deeper, largely due to the shared collective experience and challenge of physical movement.

A good friend of mine shares fifty-fifty custody of her daughter with her former spouse. When her daughter took vacations with her father, they would travel predominantly by car. They'd drive to a spot, have a look around, get back in the car, and go on their way. Her daughter would say the right things following such "adventures": "it's nice" or "so beautiful." But she lacked the ability to describe the experience with more detail, texture, or emotion. With my friend, however, the daughter would lace up her hiking books and visit places like the old-growth rainforests in the Pacific Northwest. She'd look around, glimpse the soaring canopies of the ancient trees, and dig her boots into the dirt, feeling herself momentarily part of the biodiversity in her midst. With her father, she viewed the vistas in a detached way. With her mother, she had an immersive, three-dimensional experience, using her bodily movement to connect to her environment and her parent.

In a sense, the daughter straddled the worlds of mechanization and tradition. She received traditionally nourishing and bonding physical experiences with her mother, and the nonphysical ease of modernity with her father. Of course, she resented physical experiences with her mother early on, grumbling when she returned from a hike, tired, with blisters on her feet. Like adults, children prefer ease and immediate gratification. But when this girl grows into adulthood and looks back on her family trips, I believe she'll remember the experiences with her mother most fondly and profoundly.

A Maori physical educator from New Zealand, Dr. Ihirangi Heke, draws on a similar principle of physical connection when describing how he increased the physical fitness levels of the young indigenous Maori population in New Zealand.[24] He found that telling these youths to work out in order to stave off heart disease and other afflictions fell on deaf ears. So Dr. Heke devised a different strategy, tapping into the deep spiritual connection the Maori have with their environment and the deities that, under Maori lore, form the caretakers of these environments. Dr. Heke led his students on a hike up a particular mountain that had spiritual significance. If they struggled to make it to the top due to a lack of fitness, Dr. Heke asked how they could possibly enjoy such a spiritual connection with a mountain they couldn't even summit. How was this showing respect for the mountain? These simple questions explicitly linking physical activity to spiritual awareness did much more to motivate his students to become fitter than simply exhorting them to run or pump iron.

In Maori culture, there are gods for different types of dirt, sand, wind, water, and even snow. By asking his students to experience the texture of different grains of dirt or sand, to discern the different types of snow or water, and to mimic birds or insects balancing in different winds, Dr. Heke also used movement to connect with a special environment. All the while, he increased the fitness and strength of his students without explicitly telling them to "exercise." I know I wouldn't ride my mountain bike if the sole aim was to increase my VO_2 max (the maximal oxygen amount someone can use during physical activity) or lower my risk for heart disease in thirty years' time. I *am* motivated to ride because it connects me with the warmth of the sun, a pleasing trail, or a hill summit. The spectacular views, in turn, provide a sense of exhilaration that I can share with my fellow riders or others I might meet along the way. In exploring all these connections, via my bike, I also happen to improve my aerobic fitness and reduce my risk for chronic disease. Experiences weigh more than obligations.

With these ideas in mind, my elevator pitch for how and why we should develop our physical fitness and strength boils down to this: move your body in a way that strengthens it, connects you to others, and allows you to explore your world.[25] But be smart in how you engage in such movement. Don't get your butt up at 5:00 a.m. to go for a run if you only got five hours of sleep. (Stay in bed. Really.) I'm moving (see what I did there?) away from words like "exercise" and "training" because they conjure images of grinding away at the gym, sweating your way through a timed 10K run, or spinning your way through a fitness class. While these can be good options in the right context, such a focus on fitness and exercise overlooks the importance of low-intensity movement like walking, hiking, or riding a bike and natural movements like crawling, balancing, climbing, and carrying. The latter activities all help to strengthen our bodies in ways modern life—and gyms—often cannot. Fun, playful, and restorative movements like throwing a Frisbee, playing fetch with your dog, running around with your kids, climbing a tree or a steep hill, dancing, massage, and sexual intimacy are all examples of movement that help us to connect with those we feel closest to while improving our physical health.

Given the nature and constraints of our modern lives, physical strength, rather than aerobic fitness, should form the central pillar of any structured exercise program. Resistance training, carrying, and weight lifting are all common methods of building a strong and capable musculoskeletal system. Short infrequent bursts of high-intensity activity, when added to plenty of regular low-intensity movement, give most people all the aerobic conditioning they need. I recommend varying the balance of such activities according to the seasons on the calendar and the seasons of your life.

Physical Fitness for Quality of Life

Some readers might find the discussion in this chapter frustrating. "But Dallas," they might say, "just tell me what the best exercise program is!" I really can't do that. I'm also not going to give you an easy answer like, "Just do CrossFit/yoga/jogging." Such blanket solutions, from me or others, miss the mark. As always, context matters.

We must look at physical fitness more holistically, starting with becoming more attuned to the many movement deficits we face as a society. How often do you take the escalator instead of the stairs? How often are your groceries or books delivered to your doorstep? How much time in a day do you spend in a non-seated position?

When we start asking these sorts of questions, we begin to real-ize how much we've made our world mechanical, easy, and conve-nient, essentially discouraging any physical movement. You might have rolled your eyes when I suggested you walk to your grocery store and then return home with your groceries. If so, you'll think my suggestion of taking the stairs over the escalator is also annoying. But that's a small modification we can make to get us moving and at-tuned to the presence or absence of physical movement in our lived environments. It's only when we make decisions like these that we can cultivate a healthy deviance against our society's anti-movement status quo, improving our physical health and connecting with others and our environments.

When you travel, try to make your time away more physically in-teractive. Get out of the car or tour bus, and deliberately immerse yourself in the environment. Navigate the meandering streets of Eu-rope; take off on a mountainous dirt trail and see where it leads; pitch a tent with your kids, letting them pound the stakes into the ground, and then experience the wondrousness of sleeping amidst nature. Choos-ing more interactive and physically demanding leisure activities such as these will create a richer, more enjoyable, and memorable experience. You and your children will also become more primed to exploring movement in other areas of your lives, setting the stage for bodily in-tegrity and future independence.

I witnessed the importance of cultivating lifelong strength when, during my physical therapist days in the mid-2000s, I worked with elderly patients on fall prevention and recovery. As I both observed and confirmed in the medical literature, leg strength represents one of the strongest risk factors dictating fall risk. Elderly people with higher leg strength fall less frequently and recover faster than their weaker-limbed counterparts.[26]

When elderly people fall, at least half the time it's because they trip over their pets, the edge of the carpet, the toe of the stair, or something of that nature.[27] In order to recover fast enough to regain balance, your body must have the muscular force to move your leg rapidly. People with stronger lower extremities—like legs and hips—are more likely to engage in general activity, like a solid strength-training program, that leads to stronger muscles, better balance, and therefore better reaction times (not to mention a more efficient nervous system).

It's tempting to measure people's health and fitness levels based on their muscular definition, leanness, or what they look like in a bathing suit. But as I hope I've conveyed, I'm most interested in long-term quality and enjoyment of life. And I believe that strong, durable, and resilient bodies are best able to access this. Those of us who emulate the general movements of our ancestors as closely as possible are better poised to enjoy vibrancy, health, and vigor throughout their lives, and to stay independent into old age.

I could ramble on endlessly about physical fitness. But the social connection that can arise from movement is especially important and worth focusing on. Homebound elderly who are so physically frail they cannot leave the house do not die of lack of formal exercise. They die from loneliness. Our ability to move ourselves independently connects us with other people and places. CrossFit's industry dominance and social popularity ultimately has little to do with its programming, but rather with the social bonds and connections formed when humans experience and endure something physically and mentally challenging together. As we'll explore in the next chapter, our social rootedness is perhaps the most important component of human health and well-being, eclipsing even a healthy diet and a robust physical fitness regimen.

CHAPTER FIVE

People Matter Most

On the surface, Mike has quite a full and happy life. In his late twenties, he's working his way up at a mission-driven company, on a career path that will land him, eventually, in upper management. He's also healthy, fit, and energetic, hitting the gym regularly and joining his buddies for a game of pickup basketball every few days. He's no health nut, but he's stopped partying regularly and has focused on nutrition—Paleo, to be precise. It made intuitive sense to discard those prepackaged power bars and processed staples he'd been snacking on, and to echo the eating patterns of his earliest ancestors.

And yet, all is not right in Mike's world. Somehow, he feels unmoored, and he doesn't quite know why. When he visits his parents, usually during Christmas vacation and maybe once during the summer, they ask how's he doing, and he responds with a generic, "I'm good. Everything's pretty good." If his mom presses, he steers the conversation to his career, or a new piece of furniture he's recently purchased for his apartment, or an upcoming trip. Now that he's graduated college, he no longer sees his fraternity buddies as much, and instead routinely attends after-work mixers with his colleagues. They drink beer together and decompress, keeping the talk light and easy. Deep down, however, Mike longs for more intimacy in his life—a feeling he attributes to being single. Once he finds that "special someone," maybe he'll finally feel whole.

Many people today feel lonely or disconnected. Twice as many Americans are lonelier today than they were in 1980, and that trend shows every sign of increasing. In many cases, these feelings can lead to full-blown anxiety or depression, but others of us experience them as a subtler feeling of unease. Like Mike, we shrug it off, assuming that we'll "work it out" over time. And yet, discontent about the quality and quantity of our relationships causes more harm than we realize by stressing our bodily systems. Having stronger social bonds can decrease your mortality risk by up to 50 percent, which makes strong social support and community integration just as important as smoking, drinking, obesity, and sedentary lifestyles in determining your overall health. According to former US Surgeon General Vivek Murthy, "Loneliness is a growing health epidemic."[1]

For cultural critics, the causes of our scourge of loneliness aren't all that hard to identify. With the dominance of social media and impersonal communication like texting, our social connections have increasingly lost their capacity to nourish and ground us. We might boast a multitude of "friends" or "followers," but we sustain fewer and fewer meaningful relationships. We spend time in others' company, but all too often the quality of that time is corroded as we check our phones, trying to maintain many superficial social connections all at once. Factor in other elements of modern life, such as our tendency to move from place to place seeking opportunity, or the demanding pressures many of us experience at work, and it's easy to find yourself in Mike's predicament.

In line with my seasonal model, I'd like to suggest that critiques of the impact that social media and digital technology are having on our relationships are incomplete. Social media and digital connectedness have a role in our lives, just like natural sugar has a role in our diets. Problems arise when we limit ourselves to the kinds of relationships that social media and digital technology facilitate, failing to dedicate ourselves to other kinds of relationships as well. As with food, sleep, and movement, our relationship needs are not one-dimensional. We need different kinds of relationships in their proper balance. As I'll argue in this chapter, we wind up lonely and disconnected when we fixate on what I'll call "summer" socializing, neglecting the patterns of connecting associated with other seasons. The solution, as in the other three basic areas of human health, is to dislodge ourselves from endless summer and rediscover more symbolic seasonality in how we interact with others. Only then can we achieve optimal health.

Friends for a Season

It's a cliché to observe that humans are social animals, but it's absolutely true. In his famous teachings about the hierarchy of human needs, psychologist Abraham Maslow conceived of human needs as a pyramid, with our most basic, physiological requirements for food, water, shelter, sleep, and so on residing at the bottom. As we satisfy those requirements, we can address new sets of needs higher up on the pyramid, culminating in the satisfaction of our inborn yearning for creativity and personal growth. Critically, Maslow conceived of physical and psychological safety—the products of social rootedness—as vital needs that ranked just above our baseline requirements for food, water, shelter, and sleep. After fulfilling our underlying physiological needs to keep our bodies alive, we need to see to our connection with others. Otherwise, we don't have a prayer of living happy, healthy, contented lives.

In the context of evolutionary history, our need for connection and rootedness is an old one. Absent our ability to socialize and cooperate for the greater good, large kangaroos or apes might be running the world right now, not us. During our hunter-gatherer days, individual humans were too fragile to survive on their own. We gave birth to completely helpless babies, who needed our round-the-clock care and attention. We were also terrible solitary predators, with dull teeth, poor eyesight, and insufficient physical strength and speed. Imagine a lone human duking it out on the plains with a lion—it wouldn't have been pretty. We also couldn't match the sensory prowess of most other predatory mammals, nor were we equipped to subsist on vegetation alone. As such, we found ourselves in a unique predicament: we needed to hunt and protect ourselves but lacked the raw physical capacity to do so. Poor humans. Luckily, what we lacked in physical ability we more than made up for in intelligence and the ability to cooperate.

Modern science doesn't know all the particulars of how we became social and cooperative, but I'm compelled by Yuval Noah Harari, who in *Sapiens: A Brief History of Humankind* explores the theory that around seventy thousand years ago, a cognitive revolution occurred in the human species.[2] Unlike competing species like Neanderthals, we developed a unique and wonderful ability to collect knowledge and reapply it to practical problems. While it might have taken reptiles millions of years to learn to fly, humans would come to do it over a much shorter time period through the focused, transferrable application of knowledge. And well before the Wright brothers' inaugural flights, the cognitive revolution gave us language, the ability to construct kinship and other social networks with one another, and the ability to create potential realities with our imaginations. Our cognitive abilities allowed us, for the first time, to create, share, and teach such things as technology, language, and hunting strategies within our small societies.[3]

After the cognitive revolution, we still lived in relative harmony with the land, nourishing ourselves with the plants we foraged and the animals we hunted, and enjoying meaningful connections with one another. This likely happened in a seasonally variable manner. In those ancient winters, our social worlds contracted. We invested in a few close, intimate connections, and not much else. Daylight was brief, rendering the world physically and psychologically spare. We wouldn't have risked long voyages in this cold and dark seasonal extreme, remaining instead in close, confined spaces where we enjoyed rootedness and intimacy with our core connections, our most important people. Winter also provided a space for cultivating observation, self-awareness, and introspection, a chance to know ourselves better. In the company of others, but also in our personal solitude, we became better acquainted with our hopes, dreams, visions, and future plans.

When winter finally yielded to spring, the world broadened again, becoming more expansive, exciting, and inviting. We met more people, explored more ideas, and explored different types of relationships. As we moved from spring into summer, the number of connections we made with others continued to grow, while the quality of these connections tended to become more superficial. I don't mean superficial in a negative way—I simply mean that many of our summertime connections were more like fleeting friendships or flings than lifelong connections or partnerships. Ancestral summer provided our hunter-gathering ancestors the opportunity to explore, migrate, and gather new ideas, as they also hunted extensively and gathered nature's rich bounty. We ate copious amounts of nutritious and energy-dense foods, wondered what was over that next ridge, and then actually went to find out, bringing our new friends and acquaintances along to help. Both literally and symbolically, summer was about expansion, consumption, novelty seeking, and risk-taking. It was about working hard, gathering ideas and resources, and thinking ahead with others, as we stockpiled preserved foods for the coming winter and added some extra body fat to our frames (a portable form of long-term energy storage).

As the summer sun waned and fall returned, we gradually pared down our warm-weather acquaintances. We began sifting, distilling, and picking and choosing which relationships to keep of the dozens or hundreds we might have developed during the warm-weather months. Abandoning the energetic "friend frenzy" of summer might have been difficult, but it was also part of a restorative and self-balancing pattern of expansion and contraction. As pleasant and exciting as summer socializing was, winter's quiet rootedness provided a healing time to reconnect with closer relationships, and to turn inward to ourselves. The winter home provided our ancestors with safety, belonging, rootedness, and inclusion, and an opportunity to reprioritize and reinvest in their dearest people and priorities.

The Great Separation

Our movement toward agriculture, permanent settlement, and eventually industrialization and urbanization disrupted this natural, rhythmic quality, and it also led to more social disconnection generally. We broke ourselves off from the ebbs and flows of hunting and foraging; from seasonal and migratory food sources; from the seasonal swings in temperature and exposure to precipitation (through building permanent dwellings); from the natural consequences of our extractive attitudes toward natural resources; and from an awareness of our fates as inextricably linked to the environment we inhabit. Jared Diamond's bestselling book *Collapse* outlines what happens when shortsighted humans compete for and rapidly deplete limited resources in locations such as Easter Island.[4] (Hint: it ends badly.) Our newfound imaginations led to a collective hubris, as we gradually came to believe that we were owed a biblical "dominion over the earth." Having become the most destructive and dominating species on earth, no other animal could challenge this self-indulgent claim.

So began the Great Separation. Humans began seeing themselves as separate from the earth and other living things, rather than as part of a larger, integrated whole. We no longer felt reliant on the fertility, seasons, and natural fluxes of our environment, but instead exerted control and mastery over them. We stopped syncing our movements and patterns with the earth and began directing the natural order instead. For roughly fourteen thousand years, our transition to modern civilization cemented these trends, as we devised centralized and hierarchical administrations, political structures, property ownership, systems of knowledge, densely populated communities, and divisions of labor.

New forms of community arose in cities—we had neighborhoods, occupational guilds, local religious groups. But as a whole, urbanization led to a decline in the close bonds we had formerly enjoyed with members of our tribes, and hence a sense of social unmooring and anonymity. In our burgeoning cities, we tended to spend less time with close acquaintances, and more time among strangers. Families moved from rural, multigenerational homes into atomized urban housing where they enjoyed far less community support and solidarity. When your neighbors are strangers, you lose your sense of belonging there. Absent traditional community stability, parents strained themselves, working long, hard hours to feed and care for their families. Industrialized labor further disconnected us from one another as we became increasingly specialized and isolated, losing the sense of purpose that came from providing goods and services to people we actually knew or could see regularly in a marketplace. We became obsessed with growth, efficiency, and expansion, and the "progress" we achieved only served to perpetuate our loyalty to a system premised on fracturing our ancestral interconnectedness in order to achieve more progress. But at what price? We did more work to produce less-nourishing food, and had less free time to talk, make music, dance, be playful, or simply relax.[5]

Fast-forward to modern times, when we have become stuck on what I've identified as the "summer" forms of connecting. We seek out novelty and sensation via numerous shallow and unnourishing relationships, foreclosing on the opportunity for deeper attachments. Texts and social media posts might seem social, but they really aren't. When we filter our psycho-emotional state through alphanumeric characters, we strip out the most nourishing components of human interaction. We remove human vulnerability and the subtleties of communication—nuanced social cues, gestures, touch—that can only occur in real time, with the unpredictable unfolding of complex human emotion and language. Human beings feel safe when others see us, with all our flaws, idiosyncrasies, and quirks, and love us with them all. Only the experience of being seen, known, and accepted can reduce the baseline stress that we feel and enable us to thrive. Maintaining a facade makes us feel fundamentally unsafe, since our relationships are predicated on a projected image, not an authentic expression of who we truly are. Conversely, authenticity and vulnerability, paradoxically, create opportunities for deep belonging and that critical psychological sense of safety.

Before complex language, our hominid ancestors communicated and connected largely through biological cues. They relied on facial ex-

pressions, eye contact, physical touch, hand gestures, and vocal intona-
tion to understand one another, regulate their nervous systems, and
establish safe, trusting relationships. Researchers call this experience
coregulation, which occurs when one person's nervous system interacts
with and influences another's, often outside the purview of conscious
observation.[6] In secure, loving, safe relationships, coregulation takes
the form of gentle gestures, positive expressions, loving touch, and a
relaxed or happy emotional state. In unsafe or insecure interactions or
situations, the opposite is present: mistrust, fear, defensive postures,
and a nervous system that's always on guard. Coregulation is one of
the most fundamental ways we as humans connect, beginning at birth
with the mother-child relationship and continuing onward through our
adult life and subsequent relationships and interactions.

When we become perpetually busy, distracted, and emotionally
absent, as we are in the modern world, we lack the feeling of safety
and belonging that comes with coregulation. We also miss out on those
connective experiences when we immerse ourselves in a world of two-
dimensional symbols on our digital devices. Without the opportunity
to coregulate, the rich, meaningful connection we're yearning for becomes little more than a hollow, transactional exchange of data, one
you might just as easily sustain with a highly capable computer. The
farther away we move from coregulation, the more likely we are to
forget how to do it. In her book *Reclaiming Conversation*, Sherry Turkle
poignantly observes that we are being "silenced by our technologies,"
and as a result are experiencing a "crisis of empathy."[7] Without attentive conversation, personal touch, and face-to-face interaction, we're
losing the ability to conjointly regulate our minds, bodies, and emotions, leaving us frayed at the edges and lonelier than ever.

The cultivation of closeness and intimacy requires an investment of
time. Lacking that investment, we fall into relationships by default and

convenience, like those we make with the barista at the corner coffee shop, or the people we see at work. These interactions are typically impersonal or fragile, as traditional corporate environments, for example, frame relationships as inherently competitive and hierarchical. Don't get me wrong: some of these relationships can be gratifying. A barista might remember your favorite drink in the morning and provide you with a fleeting sense of community belonging. Digitally mediated forms of communication, like text messages, also have their place. They are a great way of transmitting data ("Did you get the eggs on the way home from work?" "What time should we get together?"). But they are ultimately an impoverished and sanitized form of communication. They enable us, like Mike, to don an "everything is wonderful" facade, and to avoid the complex loneliness and even emptiness at the center of our lives.

I speak here from painful experience. Right around the time that Facebook and Twitter took off, my own career took an unexpected turn. I'd spent almost a decade in clinical practice as a physical therapist and strength and conditioning specialist, and my nerdy interest in nutrition had spilled over into many of my personal and professional conversations. I started speaking and writing about nutrition and exercise, and, along with my former partner, began traveling the country teaching nutrition seminars to enthusiastic audiences interested in improving physical performance, nutrition, and overall health.

We worked hard to grow our online audience, publishing thousands of Facebook posts, tweets, Instagram posts, blog posts, and email newsletters. I answered hundreds of online questions and responded to innumerable skeptical inquiries and overt attacks from hostile or confused strangers. During those years, I flew hundreds of thousands of miles, attended dozens of professional conferences, met incredible, inspiring people, appeared on national television many times, and . . . was really, really lonely.

I had many friends, but with my busy travel schedule and the pressure to be "just so" in the public eye, I found it hard to be truly vulnerable about my fears, flaws, and failings. If you'd asked me then, I'd have told you that my social life was incredible. I talked to dozens of friends often, met lots of interesting, successful people, and, though my marriage was crumbling, I had convinced myself that my social needs were being met. After all, how could they not be? In retrospect, I spent much of those hectic years desperately filling any spare time I had with "connections" (often online), trying to distract myself from a creeping sadness and the unsettling feeling of not truly belonging anywhere. Success, money, and recognition didn't make it better; if anything, that only increased the pressure I felt to project an image of health and happiness on my social media platforms and in my private conversations. I made the same mistakes that millions of modern, tech-savvy smartphone and internet users make every day: I confused the exchange of little snippets about my life with meaningful emotional connection.

After splitting up with my partner in 2014, I suffered depression, anxiety, and crushing loneliness, and was unclear about how to escape all of that. Once again, I distracted myself with business, traveling extensively, and learning compulsively. It took some deep soul-searching to recognize that I was, like so many others, emotionally isolated and deeply distressed. Despite writing and speaking about the perils of filtering our personal vulnerability, championing face-to-face interactions, and launching a program called More Social Less Media, I wasn't really following my own advice. Although I wasn't purposely deceiving my readers and followers, I was struggling with the same basic qualities of modern life as everyone else: chronic overstimulation, perpetual distraction, and social isolation. In other words, I lived a perpetual summer.

The problem isn't with summer itself. On a metaphorical and also literal level, summer as I've described it is about exploration, novelty, stimulation, challenge, a focus on work, acquisition, success, and "doing." The general sensation of "summer" includes the perception of scarcity (after all, winter *is* coming) despite the reality that, all around us, we see abundance, excess, and wastefulness. During the actual summer months, it's healthy and normal to go exploring (road trips!), to meet new people (neighborhood parties and barbecues), and to stay up later than usual because the sun is still out. Our problems arise when we try to maintain summer patterns of social connection *all the time*.

In effect, we become addicted to the excitement and intoxication that comes with doing and moving as opposed to sitting still and reflecting; with making quick, superficial, and usually fleeting connections with others as opposed to deeply relating and investing over time. This addiction even has a neurochemical basis to it. Social media "likes" and comments as well as advertising and other elements of modern consumer culture can give us a quick and pleasurable hit of the neurotransmitter dopamine. Famous for its role in motivation, pleasure, focus, and emotional flexibility, dopamine leaves us feeling clear-headed, euphoric, energetic, powerful, and motivated. Who wouldn't want to feel that way?

And yet, our drive to maximize these feelings leaves us unable to slow down and forge deeper connections with a few special people in our lives. With TV shows, advertisements, and pings from our smartphones endlessly seizing our attention, with traffic and media hypersexualization and noise and light pollution constantly stimulating us and delivering those dopamine hits, modern summertime drains our creativity, self-awareness, and ability to understand and empathize with others. We wind up overstimulated, overextended, isolated, and ultimately, quite lonely. It's a painful comedown.

We also wind up consuming too much. I'm speaking broadly about

our unbalanced, unconscious desire to buy, own, eat, and accumulate . . . everything. The stress of the summer bustle makes us want
more sugar, salt, fat, calories, sex, emotional validation, attention,
pleasure, and consumer goods of all sorts. Summer is about wanting
and taking action to realize our desires, but with that comes fear—the
fear of not attaining, or of losing what we have. Fear is a wonderfully
effective motivator for consumer culture, and if you've watched the
news or scrolled through your social media feed recently, you might
have felt an unsettling sense of fear. The fear of being left out or socially
rejected, the fear of not being "enough," the fear of terrorists or economic collapse or disease epidemics, and the fear of somehow being
inferior to people around us drives us to buy, lease, or borrow things
we don't need, want, or sometimes even like.

Perpetual summer nudges us into excess in other ways. We stay up
too late scrolling through Instagram or watching TV, stealing much-
needed sleep from our future selves. We spend money we don't really
have, opting in to an economic system that would leave us perpetually
indebted. We spend time commuting to work, chauffeuring kids to and
from extracurricular activities, doing yard work and housekeeping,
going to happy hour and holiday parties, and still trying to get to the
gym or go for a run so we don't gain another ten pounds like we did
last year. We're burnt out and beat down, but we can't stop. We dare
not stop. Most of us are crazy-busy (crazy + busy?), with fewer leisure
hours per day than many hunter-gatherers. Contemporary hunter-
gatherer tribes such as the Bushmen of Namibia only spend four to
five hours per day working, although it's worth noting that for many
of these tribal peoples, their "work" includes hunting, fishing, walking,
gathering nuts and wild fruit, and setting up camp, activities that, ironically, many of us more "civilized" folks might do on vacation.[8]

All of this frenzied, summer-type behavior leaves us sick. Depression, anxiety, and other dysfunctions like insomnia, mood disorders, and dementia have steadily increased since the agricultural revolution, with industrialization, urbanization, and the ever-accelerating pace of life that followed all increasing the mismatch between the natural world in which our brains evolved and the post-agricultural world that we have created.[9] Although such illnesses have no single, straightforward cause, we've spent over ten thousand years moving farther away from nature, inadvertently disconnecting ourselves from the earth, ourselves, other people, and a larger sense of purpose and meaning. It would be surprising if that didn't negatively impact human experience.

Harvard psychology professor Steven Pinker takes a brighter view of human history, arguing that the trajectory of humankind is, in fact, an upward one. As he's demonstrated, we inhabit the most peaceful era we've ever had on this planet, with far fewer deaths, illnesses, and acts of senseless violence claiming innocent lives.[10] But I wonder: What good is a long life if those lives are anxious, depressed, and lonely, and ultimately devoid of the deep meaning and purpose that comes from deep human connection? Aggregated data about large-and-ever-growing populations is little solace for those trying to understand or cope with the suffering that we individually experience.

As I'm suggesting, our crisis today isn't just a lack of deeper connections with individuals thanks to our penchant for stimulation and frenzy, but rather a lack of rootedness and connectedness in all of its forms. The farther we move away from living in smaller family clans or tribal groups, the farther we move away from a daily connection to the rhythms of the natural world, and the farther we move away from being deeply and meaningfully connected to each other, the less healthy, peaceful, and happy we humans are. Most of us sense this—we know that we are unmoored in a very big, very fast-moving world. We feel very small and, sometimes, utterly invisible and insignificant. We wonder what it's all for. We don't feel like we're contributing to anything that matters, and we lack a sense that someone "has our back" if things should go sideways.

In contrast to all the talk about social isolation's health consequences, we don't talk very much about how empty life can feel without a sense of contributing to a larger whole, whether that be extended family, a local community, or the better world we hope to leave for future generations. Working for a faceless corporation moving numbers around on a computer screen to make invisible shareholders richer doesn't do much for our sense of contribution to something that truly matters. If that last sentence makes you bristle, that's okay. I've bristled a lot at statements like this one over the years, but once I settled down, I saw the truth they contained. Simply making money for yourself or others won't leave you feeling like you've contributed much that is meaningful, just as focusing much of your attention on superficial "friend" relationships on social media won't leave you feeling seen and deeply loved.

Without a sense of contribution to something larger than yourself, you'll doom yourself to an intangible hollow feeling, and a less enriching, less healthy life.

Four Forms of Disconnection

I've painted a grim picture of modern life and (dis)connection, ranging quite far in my discussion. Let me focus my commentary a bit by identifying four forms of disconnection that I've been touching on in one form or another. As I see it, no single form of disconnection outweighs any other, but taken together they prevent us from feeling rooted, happy, and at peace. It's only when we understand how far off track we are that we can become unstuck from summer, and begin the process of reconnection.

Self

Following adolescence, most people move away from the comforts of home to explore, create, and establish roots elsewhere. They might move physically from their hometowns, or they might make a psychological break, or both. Whatever happens, they leave their own established sense of self behind to learn, grow, explore, and build.

Such behavior is both physically and psychologically healthy during the spring and summer phases of our lives, which for most people occurs during our twenties and thirties (something I explore in chapter 8). After a childhood phase in which we practice, prepare, and dream, we need to get out in the world and busy ourselves with actually doing and accomplishing our summertime projects and goals. And yet, all this action and adventure can become dangerous if we take it too far. We can lose contact with our core self, to the point where we become terrified of spending time alone and feel as if we're inherently "not enough." The longer we stay away from our home, our selves, the deeper we dig ourselves into a hole of disorientation and oblivion.

Disconnected from ourselves, many of us turn to mainstream culture for opportunities to reconnect. In recent years, as social media has influenced the way we share with and signal to one another, we've seen catchy content telling us to set boundaries around work, take our "me time," and make room for self-care and self-love. But when we finally end up scheduling that much-needed massage or taking a weekend away, the peace of mind we're hoping to attain escapes us. We walk away, wondering, yet again, what's missing.

While I certainly agree it's essential to nurture, love, and accept oneself, emphasizing bubble baths and massages, the setting of boundaries or "self-acceptance" alone isn't enough. Without complementing such activities with close observation of our very real, often unpleasant qualities, we miss the opportunity to connect with our whole selves. If we encounter an experience that challenges our positive but incomplete understanding of ourselves (divorce, major injury or illness, job loss, infidelity, eating disorders, mental health conditions), we struggle to integrate it within our larger sense of self.[11] We then fragment into two people: the person we reveal "out there" in the world, and the person we are in the shadows of our own home and minds. Such compartmentalization leaves us feeling unseen, unheard, and unaccepted by both ourselves and others. After all, if we don't show anyone who we really are, others can't know, accept, and embrace our real selves, either.

In learning to connect to our true self, we find both pride in our strengths and humility in our weaknesses. We learn to meet our own emotional needs and lovingly accept our flaws while also gently encouraging ourselves to stretch and grow. Without this type of compassionate awareness, focusing more attention on ourselves is little more than self-absorption or narcissism. Knowing, accepting, and valuing ourselves is often misunderstood or overlooked, but it's a critical component of who we bring into the world wherever we go, and a better world starts with each of us bringing forth the best versions of ourselves.

Place

As technology and urbanization press forward into seemingly endless expansion, our sense of belonging in the world we inhabit continues to diminish. For most of human history, until the last 200 years or so, we lived closer to Mother Nature's fury and bounty.[12] We understood weather patterns and seasonal oscillations. We relied on the soil's fertility and feared the raging seasonal storms. We let our feet dance naked over sun-warmed rocks and our ears bathe in the tranquil sounds of the forest. This kind of spiritual connection with our home—the dust from which we came and to which we'll return after death—is what gives us a sense of belonging to somewhere much larger and more profound than our apartments, offices, or daily grinds. Without it, we are unmoored—isolated islands within a turbulent sea of uncertainty.

Most of us recognize this need for rootedness—to have a place where we're "from" and the significance that comes with it—which is why we visit the same coffee shops, take the same route to work every day, and see the same friends every Friday night. Familiarity is calming and belonging signifies safety. Without either, the thrill of novelty quickly turns to alarm. But in a world of concrete jungles, electronic screens, and glittering drive-throughs, we've neglected and disconnected from the physical soil underneath our feet. This soil is the foundation for the homes we inhabit, the food that nourishes our bodies, and a soft, welcoming beacon for our concrete- and asphalt-weary bodies. Instead of physically grounding ourselves in natural environments, we look longingly at photoshopped pictures on the internet and fantasize about white sandy beaches and quiet mountain retreats. All of us, even those living in siren-laden cities—who proudly declare that we thrive on the noise and hustle and bustle of the city—feel deep within our bones that something is missing: the feeling of attachment, belonging, and kinship to more than just our iPhones and Facebook friends.

Offline Community

Despite the influence of our neglected geography, the most neglected form of connection in the modern world is likely that which we should be sharing with other human beings around us. Though we evolved in small tribal bands, ranging from a few dozen to a couple hundred people, we now routinely interact with hundreds or even thousands of people through digital technologies and online platforms. In ancient and modern tribal groups, both privacy and loneliness were in short supply, given the physical proximity required to successfully hunt, forage, migrate, and rear children—not to mention play, dance, sing, or otherwise socialize. We knew our fellow tribesmen intimately and they saw us in our entirety as well. Whether we liked it or not, we couldn't hide our quirks or flaws. We were seen and truly known, even if we would rather have it be different. Wearing a mask of sorts is now the online norm, and we might not even notice that we are doing it. Have you ever noticed a contrast between how dear friends or family members present themselves online versus how you know them to be? Yeah, me too. So much for the psychological safety in being deeply known and accepted.

Such tribal intimacy is no longer possible, as an inverse relationship exists between the emotional energy you can invest in any specific person and the number of people with whom you can actively maintain meaningful social relationships. In 1992 British anthropologist Robin Dunbar argued that humans can only maintain between 100 and 200 stable social relationships. He anchored this proposal in evolutionary biology and anthropology, correlating the size of the brain with the size of social groups among various primate species.[13] According to his math, humans topped out at around 150 connections that their brains could actively manage and maintain. As he then discovered, ancient villages and tribes naturally gravitated to around 150 people—after reaching that threshold, most societal groups tended to splinter off. This means that many of your 500 or 1,000 Facebook friends lie somewhere outside the neurologically limited circle of people that you can functionally maintain relationships with.[14] And if you happen to have several thousand LinkedIn contacts or Facebook friends, you probably enjoy a meaningful connection with only a small minority of them.

But let's not fixate on the actual number. I raise Dunbar's research to highlight an underlying principle of human social connection: we have a finite ability to connect with other people, and as I've suggested, most of us choose summer's quantity over the quality of relationships. We choose the titillation of summer's beach parties over the quiet comfort of winter's *hygge* (pronounced *hoo-gah*), a Danish word that loosely expresses the intimate, comfortable, cozy feeling of being present and connected, an ineffable sense of security, familiarity, reassurance, and contentedness. Ironically, as we push farther ahead into our lives of chronic summer, we crave *hygge* even more, but we're not quite sure what to do about it, since it appears nowhere to be found.

As I've noted, stripping down our deep and complex experiences to alphanumeric characters (plus emojis) on an LCD screen dramatically reduces important aspects of human communication. In terms of understanding another person, you don't get the (whole) story through text. The consequences can prove tragic. One fall evening in 2011 Sharon Seline texted back and forth with her daughter, inquiring about how she was doing at college. The daughter responded with upbeat emojis and glowing statements, just as she had broadcast on social media. And yet, that night, the daughter attempted suicide. Talk about hiding behind technology. As communications consultant Susan Tardanico wrote, commenting on this sad story in *Forbes* magazine, "Awash in technology, anyone can hide behind the text, the email, the Facebook post or the tweet, projecting any image they want and creating an illusion of their choosing. They can be whoever they want to be. And without the ability to receive nonverbal cues, their audiences are none the wiser."[15] Hiding behind our screens, we can tell whatever story we want, to ourselves and others, leaving us lonely, misunderstood, and lacking a sense of deep belonging within the interdependent, supportive web of human life.

Purpose

Although the spheres of connection I've addressed so far are not strictly hierarchical, they do build upon one another, culminating in a sense of wholeness and satisfaction in one's life. For most of his career, Maslow labeled this culmination "self-actualization," though adopted a more inclusive and expansive take during his final years, labeling the pinnacle of human expression "self-transcendence."[16] Such a reorientation underscored how our greatest sense of meaning is less focused on the self, and more on our feeling of having contributed to something outside of ourselves. The final and perhaps most transcendent form of connection—so vital and integral to our well-being—is to our sense of purpose. Most people living in the developed West tend to take a hedonistic view of happiness, regarding happiness as the maximization of pleasure. However, research increasingly shows that those who instead define happiness to include purpose and contribution enjoy better health and well-being outcomes.[17] Unfortunately, the hyperstimulating and hyper-stressing environments we inhabit cater to a never-ending pleasure quest as we seek unsuccessfully to outrun our fears, pains, and boredom by looking for quick hits of happiness everywhere we can. We, in the West, are a people of inflated expectations and, as a result, chronic disappointments. With those disappointments come a host of physical and mental symptoms that leave us feeling flat, flaccid, and in search of an elusive but still desirable panacea.[18] Nothing is ever enough. As long as we malign or ignore our deep personal purpose in favor of a list of lusts and a house in the Hamptons, indeed, nothing will ever be enough.

The Okinawans—well known for their exceptional longevity—use the Japanese word *ikigai* to refer to their purpose and meaning. Ikigai means "life worth living," and points to a belief in, and the value of contributing to, a larger purpose in life.[19] Once we frame life as something more than the perpetual pursuit of pleasure, we can notice that the endless chasing is unsustainable and that pleasure alone is unable to fill the void as we imagine it will. That was never pleasure's job in the first place. Think of the happiness/purpose contrast in the same way you think about the sugar/nutrient-dense foods dichotomy. Sugar and nutrient-poor processed foods are neither immoral nor by definition problematic, but it's easy to let our pleasurable responses to them displace a diet rich in real, vibrant, nourishing foods. Just as we should prioritize nourishing food, so, too, should we avoid letting our response to pleasure outweigh the sometimes difficult but clearly beneficial and even profound experiences of a meaningful existence such as generosity, contribution, and legacy.

After considering all the ways that we've become disconnected, hopefully this chapter hasn't left you feeling depressed about your personal future or the world in general. There are a lifetime of opportunities available for recalibrating our ways of moving through the world—places to slow down, pause, and reconnect with ourselves, important locations, other humans, and a greater sense of purpose. Even if you've operated in a summer mode of endless expansion for years or even decades, it isn't too late to start redirecting, decelerating, and embarking on a more fall-style set of behaviors (see chapters 7 and 8). In reworking our way of living, we can rediscover belonging, safety, comfort, and meaning. We can change course, not only with the ways that we connect, but also with the ways that we eat, sleep, and move. We can integrate these dynamic and enriching parts into a larger whole, a coherent system for living that is both solid and flexible, both impactful and intuitive.

Let's Keep in Touch

Have you ever stopped and wondered about the expression "let's keep in touch"? We say it all the time, but it rarely involves any actual touch. Usually, it's an expression that initiates a period of zero physical contact. "Let's keep in touch," you say to a close friend who's about to move, or to a new acquaintance you've just met. This used to mean, "Let's contact one another via telephone or handwritten letter." Nowadays, it entails following or friending someone on social media.

During my decade of perpetual summer living, which roughly corresponded to my midtwenties through my midthirties, I kept in touch with a lot of people. I relished all my spring- and summer-style friendships, using text message and social media to receive data about my "friends'" lives. Then I started reading Brené Brown, a leading authority on courage, authenticity, and vulnerability. "Owning our story can be hard," says Brown, "but not nearly as difficult as spending our lives running from it. . . . Only when we are brave enough to explore the darkness will we discover the infinite power of our light."[20] For all my friends and acquaintances, I came to realize that no one really knew me, as I'd been running and avoiding my own messy darkness for so long. I didn't have a particularly close relationship with my parents. I had friends, and some wonderful, amazing people in my life. But like Mike in the story that began this chapter, I had carefully constructed the narrative about myself that I wanted everyone to see—leaving out the uglier and messier parts.

Following this gradual realization, I took some small risks and gradually began to peel away some of the emotional armor protecting me. This happened via a return to personal, social rhythmicity, as I began a fall-like process of contraction and distillation, selecting which friendships I wanted to maintain, and which ones I could gently let go of. I then visited those most important people face-to-face or brought them to visit me. And, in the presence of people I trusted, I began revealing more intimate parts of myself.

During my midthirties, I contemplated a career change and talked openly with a few select friends about my fears of failure. It was terrifying at first, because like everyone who decides to bare their tender, deeper selves I feared abandonment and rejection. These conversations also felt awkward and contrived initially—like the feeling you get when you've not been to the gym for a long time. "This is supposed to be good for me," you think, gazing around, feeling intimidated by all the equipment, with the regular gym-goers' ease further highlighting your own sense of insecurity.

Nonetheless, I pushed through the discomfort and decided to invest more deeply in a handful of meaningful connections. And I made some people uncomfortable. "Why are you telling me this?" some people asked when I divulged personal information about myself. They weren't trying to be mean. They were simply as unpracticed at vulnerability as I was, and my efforts struck them as confronting and unsettling.

Now, at forty, I'm still learning how to prioritize and honor those closest connections amid the more spring and summer types of connections in my life. It's an ongoing process. Sometimes it manifests in my decision to decline to attend yet another big social event and say, "No, thank you," opting instead to reinvite a close circle of friends I'd recently had over to sit around the fireplace and pick up the conversation that we didn't get to finish last time. Other times, it's a decision to decline a conference in the middle of winter and stay home with my loved ones. The more I move toward self-reflection and lean into my own symbolic fall, the more inspired I am to move even farther in the direction of home, intimacy, and rootedness, and the better I feel. It feels like being exactly where I'm supposed to be for the first time in my life.

Perhaps my experience, or that of Mike, resonates with you.

Whether it does or not, the best way to get in sync socially is to start noticing your behaviors. Take a moment and reflect: Do you feel like you have a tribe? Do you feel profound, deep belonging with a close circle of people who know your deepest secrets, fears, and dreams? If not, is this because you haven't revealed these personal details to others, or because you don't know them yourself?

To know ourselves, we must know our history. In other words, prior to introspection, I recommend retrospection. Examine your childhood experiences and past romantic relationships. What tendencies do you notice? What are your strengths when interacting with others? Where do you tend to go off-track? If you suffer from anxiety, depression, obsessive-compulsive disorder (OCD), or any number of similar experiences that impinge on your mental health, and you haven't sought help, do it now. Find a therapist. Start moving toward a healthier, happier you. And go easy on yourself. It's a common experience not to know yourself, given how distracting the outside world is. It's also common to have lived in a chronic summer social mode for a long time, neglecting self-knowledge and intimacy with others. Almost all of us are off-track here, and we would all benefit from reclaiming this part of our lives.

Whether you start meditating, begin journaling, seek counseling, or do something vulnerable and begin to share deeper parts of yourself with a group of intimate people (or anchors; see chapter 6), you'll inevitably slow down. You'll do fewer things. Or to put it in the terms of my seasonal model, you'll move away from summer kinds of behaviors and approach a fall or winter mode. Getting out of summer—no matter what the actual season is—and slowing down is the only way you'll ever acquire self-knowledge and then develop and prioritize meaningful connections with others. So, if you are ready, reinvest in your closest relationships, say yes to fewer big social engagements, and make a much deeper, personal investment in yourself.

But you need not stay in winter mode forever, either. Tuning yourself to seasonal change and rhythmicity is vital. You need balance, variety, and differing perspectives, and seasonality provides these elements. In chapters 7 and 8, I go into extended detail about how to strike that balance. But first, as we'll explore in the next chapter, there's a bit of a catch.

One of the great paradoxes of human life and of the physical world is that oscillation itself must be rooted in a fixed point, in a place of permanence. Though oscillations ought to govern our eating, exercise, and sociability patterns, there remain core pillars of our existence—also related to nutrition, movement, sleep, and connection—that must remain unchanged throughout our lives. These core foods, sleep habits, everyday movement patterns, and relationships nourish and anchor us, serving as beacons and safe harbors, grounding and protecting us amid life's turbulence and tumult, and putting us in a position to accommodate the seasonal changes we so desperately need to live life to the fullest.

PART TWO

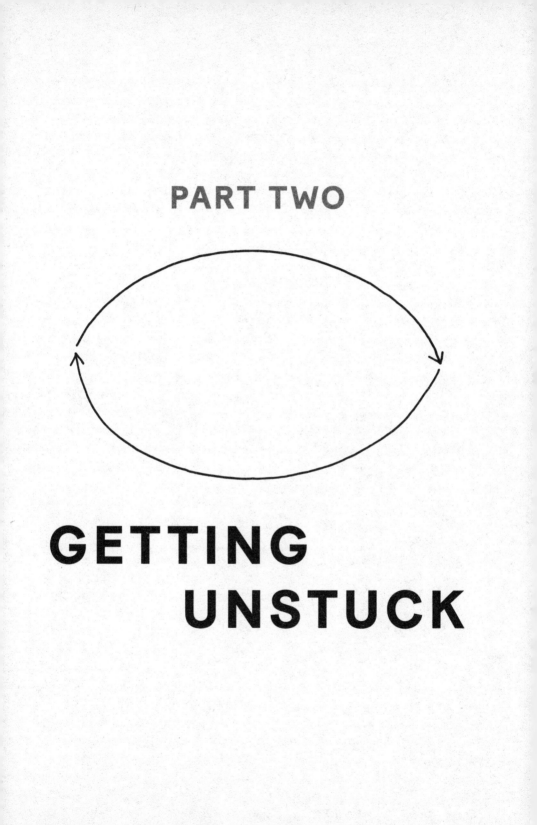

GETTING
UNSTUCK

CHAPTER SIX

Anchors

n 2012, before a small group at the Ancestral Health Symposium at Harvard, I unveiled my seasonal health model for the first time. On a 48 x 48-inch poster, I depicted all four seasons on a large clockface, with three concentric circles representing sleep, food, and movement (social connection hadn't occurred to me as central yet). This complicated poster must have struck observers as a bit daunting.

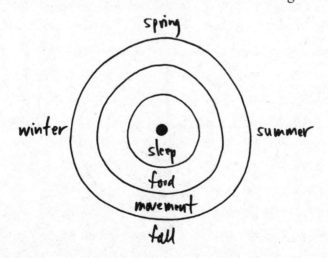

As I explained to conference-goers, sleep, diet, and movement—three pillars of human life and my model's core lifestyle variables—should properly oscillate throughout the year, with the height of summer defining one extreme and the depth of winter another. Sleep, I hypothesized, should be shorter over summer, with the early sunrise and late sunset, and more extensive during winter's prolonged periods of darkness. Our diet, I argued, should oscillate from higher-carbohydrate and lower-fat content in the summer (with fruits, vegetables, and honey available) to lower-carbohydrate and higher-fat foods over winter (with fatty animal products more plentiful). The lighter, warmer days of summer provide occasions, I said, for longer and lower-intensity movements like hiking, brisk walking, and so on. Winter's shorter days, by contrast, lend themselves to brief, higher-intensity bursts of activity.

I described how our society had resisted the less immediately gratifying seasonal oscillations of the cooler months, as we'd become locked into perpetual summer. To help convey my ideas, I made the presentation interactive, moving the poster's various clock hands to demonstrate the common lifestyle/seasonal mismatches we've considered in this book, such as eating a winter diet (low carb) while doing summer exercise (chronic cardio) and getting consistent summer sleep (up early, down late), irrespective of the actual season.

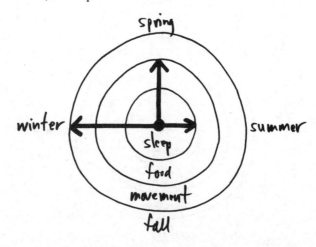

What I didn't realize at the time was that my seasonal model missed something crucial: an anchor point. For all my emphasis on rhythms, seasons, and cycles in this book, you could easily conclude that human beings exist—ideally—amid permanent change and flux. Today, I know differently. While all the seasonal and lifestyle oscillations I've described in past chapters are crucial, so, too, are the fixed points—the constants—that ground them. Oscillation itself depends on fixity. A pendulum, after all, swings on a fixed point that anchors and enables the instrument's oscillation. A teeter-totter moves up and down on a fixed central axis. A wheel revolves around a central fixed axle. When navigating a voyage, we begin with a fixed geographical location or map, and then chart our movements relative to that position.

The same principle holds for seasonality. Amid life's variability, we must maintain stable, year-round sources of dietary protein, very dark nights and light-filled days, functional movements like walking, lifting, and carrying, and a close group of intimate connections. These dietary, sleep, movement, and social requirements don't change seasonally, and allowing for them makes my seasonal model less dizzying and daunting. Rather than trying to juggle multiple variables in a life that perhaps already feels chaotic and overwhelming, you can instead focus on anchoring yourself in a stable set of unchanging practices. Oscillation is important, but I now realize that these anchors—the constants—form the most critical linchpin of my seasonal model. You need to get these right before you focus on the oscillation.

Return to Ritual

I first realized the importance of anchoring specific lifestyle components after hearing my friend Baya Voce's 2016 Salt Lake City TEDx Talk called "The Simple Cure for Loneliness."[1] Baya is an expert on human connection, serving as chief strategy officer of Secret Experiences, a design company that helps organizations create meaningful and lasting experiences. Human connection also suffuses her life and purpose. It's why she joined a reality TV show in her early twenties, and why she and I met nearly weekly for a time to explore that topic.

To overcome the epidemic of loneliness that afflicts our digitized, disconnected world, Baya proposes ritual, not in the sense of a religious or spiritual exercise, but of an activity that anchors us socially. Ritual is so powerful because it's repeated action plus intention, says Baya. When these two are combined, ritual becomes ingrained just like habits do.

Baya and her friends decided many years back to build ritual into their workweeks. Every Monday night, they pulled on their leggings and gathered at one person's house, poured a glass of rosé, and piled on the couch to talk. Think of the couch as the metaphorical fireplace around which our ancestors once gathered. On many Mondays, the women arrived excited, ready to share news about their careers, families, and relationships. Other times, they were dispirited, and sometimes devastated, sharing painful details about miscarriages and divorces. Through grief and celebration, however, the ritual remained a touchstone, allowing everyone a fixed point from which to navigate their connections, both inside and outside the group.

It took a moment of extreme crisis for Baya and her friends to recognize their ritual's full meaning and power. The year was 2016, and they were on vacation together in France. Having arrived in Paris for the first time, Baya was charmed by the city's iconic shutters and windowsills as well as the sweet smells wafting from the bakeries. She admired France's ritualized mealtimes, during which people ditched their electronic devices and spent several hours enjoying a meal and connective conversation with close friends and family. But the warm glow of novelty and happiness ended suddenly when Baya and her friends arrived in the city of Nice. It was Bastille Day, and, in a horrifying terrorist attack, a man had just driven his truck into a crowded street, killing eighty-four people. Amid the fear, anxiety, tragedy, and loss, it would have been easy for residents of the city to retreat to their homes, seeking safety and solace in private. But not twelve hours after the tragedy, storefronts and restaurants had opened their doors, welcoming people in to congregate and connect while partaking in France's cherished mealtime ritual.

Inspired by what they saw, Baya and her close friends likewise returned to the anchor that had served them so well. That summer night, thousands of miles from home, they went back to their apartment, got into their comfy clothes, poured some rosé, and piled all together onto the couch. "So my invitation to you today is simple," Baya said during her presentation, reflecting on this ritual. "Don't do something new. Find something you're already doing with your friends and families, your intimate relationships, or within your communities, and do that thing over and over and over again. Do it with intention. Do it during the good times and do it during the mundane. So when the inevitable emotional storms hit, you have your ritual to go back to. You have your very own anchor of connection."

Listening to Baya's talk, I asked myself the same question I explored in chapter 5: How did we as a species become stuck in an epidemic of loneliness? Why do we lack these grounding, core connections that rooted our ancestors, and that still root residents of the Blue Zone societies, who experience exceptional longevity and above-average happiness? My thoughts turned to the discipline of psychology and to attachment theory, which I'd found helpful as I'd wrestled with depression and a lack of meaningful relationships. Popular in the psychotherapy community for decades, attachment theory holds that secure connections—what I call "anchor connections"—are critical for human psychosocial health.

We seek these profound, anchoring connections early in life, typically from a parent. If we experienced parental security in our own childhoods, we move through life with greater physical and emotional security; if we didn't, we sometimes develop insecure attachment styles, avoiding others or anxiously attaching to them.[2] Either way, our desire for this firm social base—whether we received it as children or not—remains deep-seated and persists into adulthood. To attain psychosocial health and well-being as adults, we must embrace these desires and attach (or to use my vocabulary, anchor) ourselves to close family, romantic partners, parents, children, or friends. They alone can provide us a consistent, secure base from which to navigate an uncertain world.

Though we can't be certain about how attachments functioned among our ancestors, we can infer that they enjoyed rooted connections, and that such bonding and solidarity provided neurological and psychological advantages. If ancestral babies didn't receive adequate amounts of the hormone oxytocin from their caregivers, for example, deeply bonding them during early infancy, they would have been less likely to thrive.[3] Something analogous held true for the tribe as a whole. A strong man with great hunting prowess, an especially observant female forager, someone with especially strong intuitions: primitive societies had a place for all of these different people, assigning them roles relating to food acquisition or, in the case of someone gifted with insights about human existence, perhaps the role of shaman or religious guide (that is, someone who stood at the intersection of the physical and spiritual worlds, and could access unseen forces). This diversity of characteristics, preserved in groups, allowed our ancestors to better mobilize in times of hardship and survive. Because tribespeople were closely rooted to one another, because they bore solid attachments to one another, the group stood a better chance of surviving with more varied skills and abilities.

The same principle should apply in a modern context, where resources, talents, physical strengths, and intelligence aren't equally distributed among us all. As social animals, we don't have the capacity to go it alone, nor should we want to. Our best hedge against life's uncertainty and difficulty is a core group of intimate acquaintances. One of the hallmarks of anchor connections is that they are deep-rooted, predictable, and reliable—imperfect, perhaps, but stable. As my friend Katy Bowman, whose work on biomechanics I explored in chapter 5, has observed, many people around the world—especially where I live in Utah—stockpile food, water, weapons, and gold in case of apocalyptic catastrophe. But as Katy commented in personal conversation, she doesn't do that. Instead, she described a different strategy: handpicking a small group of people to serve as a capable, resilient safety net for tough times.

Katy seemed to echo Baya's thinking; both treat people as our most valuable resource. They are right. You might have millions of dollars in the bank, but what happens when you receive a cancer diagnosis? What happens when you're emotionally stressed or lonely or riddled with anxiety? No money, power, or influence can ease those heartaches. Only the emotional support of those psychologically and emotionally proximate to us, the people to whom we give access to the deepest parts of ourselves, can help. To prepare ourselves for life's uncertainties, we must develop sleep, eating, movement, and social anchors. Anchors give us something to hold onto when the storm rages around us.

Security and Stability

You might still be thinking: Dallas, here you are, deep into this book, arguing that the starting point for living wilder, more rhythmically attuned lives must be our fixed anchors. What gives?

Anchors have always informed my thinking, even when I didn't realize it. On reflection, the Whole30 program is an anchoring framework for our food selection and meals. It asks participants to create a dietary anchor—a base diet lacking processed food products, legumes, grains, dairy, added sugars, and other known sources of bodily inflammation. Once that dietary reference point is established, people can build a broader, more individualized dietary framework, which hopefully includes some oscillation, like eating seasonally.

Most of us already have well-established anchors in our lives, otherwise known as our habitual behaviors. Chances are, your alarm goes off at the same time every workday, whether you are ready to wake up or not. You might have attached yourself to your favorite cereal as a way to start your day. You might connect with the same social media accounts, via the same device, as you eat your cereal. And your morning commute or workout might unfold along the same route every day that you do it.

All too often, however, we're anchoring to the wrong things, and as a result, we oscillate incorrectly (or not at all). We anchor to late nights and alarm-clock mornings, shifting to the occasional early night and natural wake-up. We anchor to highly processed, predominantly refined carbohydrate foods throughout the year and shift to the occasional nutrient-dense, high-quality protein meal when our bodies start yelling at us about it. We anchor to our habitual cardio exercise and shift to the occasional strength-training session in the weight room or in the garage. We anchor to countless hours of image and content creation for our superficial social media connections and "community" and shift to occasional real-life interactions with friends, loved ones, and community members.

We've constructed and accepted these environments, and the short-term dopamine rewards they give us powerfully reinforce them. Sure, you're tired and a good night's sleep is exactly what you need.

But the allure of your social media feed or the TV series you are binge-watching is far more powerful than your desire for a good sleep. If you started an Instagram account to promote nourishing, seasonal, and locally grown whole foods, but you get three times as many likes for posting photos and recipes for cupcakes and grain-free cookies, guess what you're going to keep doing?

That's not your fault, given the powerful forces anchoring us to the status quo. Legions of trained psychologists, sociologists, and behavioral analysts have carefully engineered social media platforms to play on our insecurities and hold our attention for as long as possible. The entire modern "attention economy" is based on extracting time from our lives, so that businesses can benefit economically from it. The visual design, colors, time delays, and notification pings play on our fears of missing out and our deep-seated desires to avoid rejection or exclusion from social norms. Social media has taken a natural human instinct— the comparison of ourselves to others—and flipped it. Instead of comparing ourselves to our fellow tribesmen, whose collective intimacy afforded us little privacy but also little loneliness, social media encourages us to maximize our strengths and minimize our weaknesses. We then scroll through feeds in which we compare ourselves, in all our flaws, quirks, and dreams, to others' carefully curated and distortive self-representations. That's an apples-to-oranges comparison.

Although we increasingly recognize the toxicity and hollowness of such interactions, it's still scary to limit, let alone reject, this fast food of connection. It's just like the painful transition from summer to fall that I've described throughout this book. Altering your current, maladaptive fixed anchor points and following a new, seasonal, cyclical path is tough. Before I outline my framework's key anchor points, let's acknowledge the constraints and limitations we face in making such changes. You might be a shiftworker (or a night owl). You might have a long daily commute. You might live alone, with few close, real-world connections. You might support a tribe of hungry teenagers on a limited budget. In these and other ways, your current life might prompt you to adopt unhealthy behaviors, but they are familiar, and grounded in routines. Breaking these habits for something novel, different, and healthier might seem daunting.

For most of my life, I struggled with what attachment theory would term an insecure attachment style. Because I didn't form close attachments as a child, I was uncomfortable with intimacy and vulnerability in my adult relationships, and I would distance myself and shut down whenever family, friends, and romantic partners asked me about my emotions. But once I developed the seasonal model and understood the deep value of intimacy, I realized that I was electing to stay in a place of social isolation and loneliness, and that this was ultimately self-defeating and unhealthy. At that point, I had to make my model pragmatic and not simply theoretical. It's one thing to write about the importance of close, intimate anchor connections and quite another to embark on a journey to actual intimacy. When I finally found the courage to become more vulnerable with others, I experienced profound self-transformation. One of the reasons I wrote this book was to offer readers an intellectual framework for improving their lives, and perhaps a catalyst to take that first step.

Since breaking unhealthy attachments usually means working against common societal and cultural norms, please approach this in a spirit of experimentation and creativity. Consider the primary anchor points I describe below for the four areas of health, and embrace the ones you feel you can integrate into your life straightaway. When those are well embedded, build from there. If you are in a position to make wholesale changes, trialing them, say, for one lunar cycle, fantastic. Your context, however, might allow you to make only one incremental change over the course of a season. That's fine too. The goal isn't to pull off a quick, total, but potentially short-lived perfection. It's to make lasting and sustainable changes, season after season. And that might mean taking your time.

Anchor Points for Sleeping

Our sleep-wake cycles, the centerpiece of our circadian rhythm, should in theory sync with the changing light-dark cycles across the seasons. The changing lengths of day and night across the year should drive the oscillation of our sleep-wake times. This means that those of us living farther from the equator will experience greater fluctuations in our sleep patterns throughout the year. I can well imagine the reaction I would get from most readers if I were to say, "Anchor your sleep oscillations to the physical sunrise and sunset. Wake up at 5:00 a.m. (or earlier) in summer, and after 9:00 or 10:00 a.m. in midwinter."

From a health perspective, there would be little wrong with this guidance. But, of course, our modern world doesn't operate like this, and there are practical limits to how far we can opt out of our society's asynchronous norms. A pragmatic approach to improving sleep is to create anchor points around our sleep environment (the inner sanctum of which is our bed and bedroom) and around some of the rituals and habits that impact our sleep quality and duration.

Think about your sleeping environment, starting in your bedroom and moving outward from there. There is a strong chance that many of you have your bedroom lit up like the Las Vegas Strip. You have phones, laptops and tablets, and perhaps worse, large television screens beaming into one of the smallest areas of your home, most likely with the main lights turned off. With low ambient light, your pupils open wide, taking in significant high-intensity blue-spectrum light from these screened devices. This leads to light-induced melatonin suppression, and subsequent disruptions to your sleep quality and quantity.

We therefore must anchor our bedrooms to darkness. To do so effectively, our bedrooms must become analog rather than digital. Yes, I've heard it before—you can't make your bedroom analog, because you need your phone as an alarm clock. If you really need an alarm clock, buy a cheap analog travel device. If you absolutely cannot do that, create your alarm clock profile, put the phone in flight mode, and then place it under your bed or on the other side of the room. Do all of this before heading to bed so that you maintain your bedroom as a dark space.

Perhaps you need your phone in your room because you are on call, or the kids are out at night and you have told them to call you in case of emergency. Fair enough. Instruct such contacts to call rather than message you. Put your entire phone in dark/night mode, dim the screen to the maximum allowable limit, and disable notifications from every app. In short, transform your smart and bright minicomputer miracle machine into a dim, dumb phone. Or, get a cheap landline and circulate that number to loved ones who agree only to use it for emergencies.

If your phone doesn't need to be in your room, remove it. The same goes for electronics larger than a phone. You have no need for a computer or television in your bedroom. If you enjoy watching TV to relax before going to bed, fine, but do this in another room. If your partner wants to watch television in bed and won't remove it from the bedroom, then some tough love might be required—maybe one of you needs your own bedroom.

Recall that quality restorative sleep is predicated on darkness at night and bright natural light exposure early in the day. Irrespective of the time of day you awaken, or of the season, healthy sleep-wake cycles require you to get your eyes outside into bright light for as long, and as frequently, as possible. From the time you wake up, look for opportunities to increase your bright natural light exposure. Open your home's window blinds as early as possible and delay wearing sunglasses. Increase your time outside as much as possible before you head indoors (between parking your car and entering your workplace building, for example). Take your breaks either as close as possible to a window with bright light streaming in or, better yet, go outside. I discussed this idea with a die-hard exercise enthusiast who now does as many of her morning workouts as possible outdoors, even trekking the equipment she needs out into the parking lot. As she's reported, this has enhanced her sleep quality, her ability to recover from injury, and her performance strength and quality.

A light-meter app can come in handy. Most smartphones have a built-in light meter controlling everything from screen brightness to camera settings. Downloading an app gives you the ability to access this feature and to quantify the amount of light you receive, allowing you to either increase or decrease the light intensity to which you are exposed. I personally use an app called Lux Light Meter. Creating an awareness of how bright different environments are really helps to shift behaviors.

Even with the research I've done and the awareness I now have, I'm always surprised at just how different indoor and outdoor environments are. If it is 500 lux in your office, but 50,000 lux outside, then it is one hundred times brighter outdoors than indoors. Conversely, at night, if it is less than 5 lux outdoors, but 500 lux in your lounge room, then it is one hundred times brighter indoors than out. Your ultimate goal should be to decrease the magnitude of difference between each environment and anchor those exposures as best you can. In an ideal world, morning's bright light would awaken you from your slumber and evening's sundown initiate your sleep. But in this imperfect world, a little technology can help anchor us too.

My final recommendation for improving sleep-wake cycles and circadian rhythms is to anchor your sleep and waking times across the week. Most people understand the jet-lag effects of traveling across time zones, yet they often fail to recognize that varying your sleep-wake times (often by a few hours) from one day to the next elicits a similar jet-lag effect (commonly referred to as social jet lag). If you have ever experienced jet lag, you'll know that even if you do manage to get sufficient sleep, you will often feel tired, lethargic, and out of sorts, highlighting the effect circadian rhythm disruption (independent of sleep time) has on our energy and well-being.

Try to establish anchoring routines around a set wake-up time (preferably a natural wake-up time rather than an alarm-induced one) and a set bedtime, along with habitual ways of winding down prior to climbing into bed. For those whose waking and sleep times change according to their work schedules, such routines hold even more importance, as these secondary zeitgebers can help your body to recalibrate to new sleep-wake routines. This in turn helps to improve, as much as possible, a less-than-ideal situation when it comes to our daily rhythms.

Anchor Points for Eating

In chapter 3, I outlined key anchors and oscillations for food and nutrition, the fundamentals of which I captured in my elevator pitch for how I eat. To jog your memory, here it is again:

> Eat naturally occurring and minimally processed foods like meats, eggs, vegetables, and fruits. Choose these whole, nutrient-dense foods over packaged, processed foods, which are often nutrient poor but calorie dense. Food quality is important—a concept that includes where food

comes from (local), how it was raised or grown (humanely; organic), and its overall environmental impact.

Aim for well-balanced nutrition—this means you must eat a diet of predominantly unprocessed plant-based foods, anchored by appropriate amounts of quality animal-based protein foods. This balanced combination of plants and animals provides you with all the nutrients you need, including all the proteins, carbohydrates, and fats naturally inherent in these food groups. How you eat—the social and cultural aspects of food and nutrition—is just as important as what you eat.

From this dietary approach, we can infer several anchors that endure across the seasons. I encourage anyone first embarking on a seasonal journey to start with the qualitative aspects of their meals and how they eat. Meals with quality whole foods represent the starting point in a good nutritional journey. I encourage three full meals per day, each of roughly the same size. Since most people begin with a small or absent first meal, and save an enormous meal for the end, this is a departure from common patterns. Each of these meals should take advantage of the protein leverage effect I detailed in chapter 3, anchored by a source of high-quality protein (preferably animal protein) roughly the size of your hand (an ideal approximation that scales to different body sizes).

You can select other foods to accompany this protein anchor based on seasonal availability. What is available seasonally should drive your food selections. Take a broad view, and regardless of the oscillating parts of your meals, anchor your diet to whole, single-ingredient (for the most part), minimally processed foods in each meal. This allows you to aim for a quality protein intake of approximately one gram per pound of lean body weight (your total body weight minus the weight of your total body fat), and will have transformative effects on you, your family, and your community. It sounds too simple, but it's also massively impactful.

Anchor Points for Movement

In the West, where most of the population is sedentary, I'm not as picky about the particulars of regular physical movement. If your major seasonal mismatches include circadian rhythm disruption, poor sleep, and inadequate nutrition, I wouldn't unduly focus on physical activity patterns. But if you can focus on improving your physical activity, begin by seizing every opportunity for incidental movement, embracing inconvenience, and rebelling against efficiency. Take the stairs. Walk more. Commute to work on your bike. Hand-grind your coffee rather than using a machine.

If changing habits in these areas is too difficult, then try working in purposeful bouts of exercise. The best exercise and activity programs encompass the three M's: (Joint) Mobility; Muscle (Strength); and Mitochondria. Mitochondria are the microscopic power plants of our cells, and they need to function well if we are to be able to use food energy efficiently. We need a routine, preferably a daily one, that can guide our joints through their full range of movement, keeping them and their associated structures strong and mobile. We should also incorporate movements that allow for safe yet progressively high weight loads across the most fundamental of human movement patterns: squatting, hip hinging, lunging, pushing, pulling, and carrying. Finally, we should incorporate motions that nourish our mitochondria, the key energy-producing and regulating apparatus of our cells.

Traditionally, experts have considered cardio or endurance-type exercise (exercise with elevated and sustained heart rates) most beneficial to improving mitochondrial health. More recently, researchers and professionals have come to understand that short bouts of high-intensity efforts (such as interval training) elicit similar benefits. Strength training can also improve mitochondrial density and efficiency while enhancing joint mobility.[4]

If pressed to recommend one method of structured activity to anchor you throughout the year, I would suggest weight lifting, either as a stand-alone activity or as a complement to other functional strength movements like calisthenics. You could achieve strong outcomes, for example, by anchoring to regular yoga classes; adding CrossFit, Starting Strength, or some other form of basic strength training; and boosting your mitochondria with regular walking and general activity. Yoga, Pilates, or body-weight resistance exercises, performed at home, provide sufficient loading to build strength for nearly everyone, especially people just beginning their movement journeys. Bottom line: generating physical strength must be a consistent focus across time rather than a seasonally variable add-on.

Anchor Points for Social Connection

I've spoken of Baya Voce's TEDx Talk and of the importance of anchor connections. Such anchors are our safe harbors. People constantly ebb and flow in our lives, but amid these seasonal and lifetime social oscillations, we must invest in and nurture the core connections that offer us the greatest sense of belonging and community.

We must also take steps to remain rooted in a sense of place. We often refer to our anchor places as *home*—our physical residence, rented or owned, that contains our belongings. A place of shelter, safety, and security. Think of the violation we experience when someone enters our home who is otherwise unwelcome. Home can also take on spiritual dimensions. I am Canadian by birth but have been an American resident for most of my adult life. Ask where home is for me—which land resonates most emotionally for me—and for all the beauty of Utah (where I currently live) and the many US states and countries I have visited, I'll tell you my true homeland is British Columbia.

No matter where our life journey takes us, and no matter how many decades we've spent moving about during the "summer," expansion phases of our lives, we all do best when we have a sense of place—either a physical or spiritual home—to which we can return. This might be a physical address, a homeland, or some other anchoring space, like a piece of furniture with your photographs and plants. In today's freelancing and gig economy, many of us have inconsistent work environments, leaving us physically and psychologically unsettled. We might work at coffee shops and forgo our own vehicles for car-sharing apps like Uber. Even so, we can still find ways to enjoy anchoring spaces in our lives.

At my regular coffee shop, I have a favorite spot to sit and work. When I arrive and someone else is at my favorite table, I become almost visibly affronted. That's because, in some small way, my physical and psychological connection to this coffee shop corner provides me a sense of belonging, just like my anchor social connections. You might have carved out a similar area in your home or workplace. Or maybe you regularly walk in a park near your home when you need to clear your head or have a favorite spot you and your family return to when camping. Maybe your town, state, or country provides an anchor for your overseas deployments in the military. These are all options. Make a mental note of these places/spaces, the feelings and connection you have with them, and why you always return to them.

Connections to people and places ultimately provide us a deeper understanding of and connection to ourselves and our personal sense of purpose. In reciprocal fashion, such self-connection helps us develop deeper connections with people and places. As I recently confirmed with a close friend, our core anchor connection must be to ourselves and our purpose in life. My friend sells health insurance and routinely finds herself emotionally involved with her clients (supporting them in either accessing adequate coverage or in making a claim). As she described to me, this tendency, combined with her husband's health problems and her concern for the health of her adult daughters, all added stress to her life. When I encouraged her to prioritize her own well-being over her husband, daughters, and clients, she felt anxious about it, worrying that she would be letting these others in her life down.

After guiding her through a process to elicit her values, we found that caring served as her primary life value, defining her sense of purpose. She cared that her clients had the optimal insurance coverage to meet their health needs. She cared that their claims were met. She cared about her husband's health and would do anything to prevent it from deteriorating. She cared about her daughters and wanted them to avoid the ill health she saw in many of her clients. Understanding this, I told her that if she let her own health and well-being deteriorate, she wouldn't have the capacity to care for others in her life. That did it— something clicked.

Prior to our conversation, my friend's sense of purpose and connection to self was solely contingent on the connections she had with others in her life. Such a tendency is widespread, especially in the modern West, where we tend to view people as either altruistic or selfish.[5] In an attempt to demonstrate that we fall on the correct side of this binary and are generous, we sacrifice ourselves, purportedly for the good of others, and often at great expense to ourselves. I find it unhealthy to occupy an extreme at either end of the altruism/selfishness binary. To create healthy attachments, we must extend generosity to ourselves *and* to our deep anchor connections. Once my friend realized that all the caring she showed others should extend to her, she developed a richer internal world, and more capacity to experience self-love, self-respect, self-esteem, self-appreciation, and self-compassion. This in turn enabled her to be more present and emotionally available with other people. It's admirable and noble to care for others and place them first. But we must extend such deep investment, generosity, and compassion to ourselves as well.

Setting Your Anchor

People. Places. Purpose. Dietary protein. Functional movement. Robust sleep routines. These are the important anchors that travel with us along life's journey. They are an intentionally and unavoidably tangled web. Food connects us to people. It can connect us to places too. Food can fuel our physical, emotional, and mental energy so that we can achieve a sense of purpose. Dietary nourishment reduces our reactivity to stress, which makes us more receptive to, and more affiliative with, those around us. Insufficient sleep alters the default settings of our brain from pro-social to antisocial. When we're exhausted and sleep deprived, we lose our connection with people and places; we lose our sense of purpose (or we lack the emotional bandwidth to explore our purpose in the first place, leaving us bewildered and generally uninspired). Physical capacity allows us to move freely and confidently, taking us toward people and places. It allows us to walk up the mountain or to swim in the sea or lake or visit a friend in another country. And perhaps most notably, fostering our most important relationships anchors us so that we can more gracefully and successfully weather life's storms. People provide stability, and often serve as the greatest catalysts for feeling a deep sense of rootedness in and contribution to a larger whole. These anchors are beautifully and profoundly interconnected.

It still might seem paradoxical that anchors serve as the basis for our rhythmicity. But that's precisely how the natural world works. The universe is perpetually ebbing and flowing. Its tempests and storms are dynamic and oscillatory. Yet such dynamism exists within a very predictable framework. There are 365¼ days a year—that never changes. Every lunar month contains the same number of days. Gravity is very predictable. If this all sounds overwhelming and too abstract, don't worry. There are a few bedrock, foundational things you can do to tiptoe your way into a healthier lifestyle.

Maybe you are already experimenting with eating seasonally, or maybe not. Either way, you likely aren't approaching rhythmicity in a coordinated, synchronized, or comprehensive way. And that's okay. The anchoring principles we've examined will provide you with a baseline— the biggest return on investment for your personal health and happiness. When life gets crazy and you become stressed or lose your job or get an illness or suffer an unexpected death or end of a family relationship, you'll have these anchors. Setting anchors is the first step in establishing a healthy life foundation. But before we can begin living in a seasonally oscillating manner, firmly anchored in our four lifestyle variables, we must first compensate for our extensive period of chronic summer living. As I describe in the next chapter, we're all due for a prolonged period of healing—we all need a fall pivot and a therapeutic winter.

CHAPTER SEVEN

Pivot to Heal: Fall and Therapeutic Winter

After completing my master's degree at the age of twenty-two, I married my college sweetheart, started my career as a physical therapist, and began living a fairly conventional American life. At that time, I was poorly equipped to handle the pressure of student loan debt and the psychological stress of "adulting" and found that I felt better when I exercised. Hard. Often. I crammed a lot of competitive volleyball, running, climbing, strength training, and Olympic weight lifting into my twenties. Friends and strangers admired my physique and athleticism (which only encouraged me to do more training), but underneath it all, I had occasional inklings that all wasn't well in the henhouse. Whenever I was unable to work out, such as when I was nursing an illness or injury, or when I was simply away at a conference, I'd become anxious, jittery, and irritable. I also had a nagging shoulder injury that stubbornly refused to heal, but that I also stubbornly refused to rest. Addictions are powerful things.

As I "matured" into my later twenties, I slowly realized that I had developed a psychological dependence on exercise, using hard training to deal with a life that didn't feel deeply satisfying. I was using intense exercise to self-medicate and deal with financial stress, the lack of emotional connection and nourishment in my marriage, a lack of deeply gratifying social connections, and the extended illness and eventual death of my father from pancreatic cancer (which left me grieving and abruptly confronted by my own mortality). I also used exercise to quell my own anxiety and insecurity about my self-identity and my life's larger direction and purpose. Not surprisingly, the people I often hung around with behaved similarly, so there wasn't anyone with healthier habits to highlight my dysfunctional choices.

What I know now is that my story isn't unusual. Many of us seek a reprieve from modern environmental stressors and our chronic summer lifestyles in workaholism, alcohol, food, sex, recreational drug use, compulsive shopping, and, yes, even exercise. In the case of intense or prolonged exercise, the structural and metabolic stress triggers hormonal responses (adrenaline and cortisol) as well as the release of feel-good endorphins. For our hunter-gatherer ancestors, these endorphins helped increase our physical pain tolerance, enabling us to fight or flee from dangerous predators and threats. But in the modern world, we've unconsciously repurposed these natural painkillers to manage other types of pain and stressors, like loneliness, social rejection, financial pressure, feelings of inadequacy, and lack of deep connection with our family, friends, and romantic partners. This works because the brain circuits involved with perception of physical pain also light up when we experience social rejection. That is, being excluded or breaking up *hurts*, so self-made painkillers are a convenient and effective way to deal with that. The problem, of course, is that the net effect of excessive exercise (when it's long and/or very intense) is to add even more stress to an already overloaded system.

As I got closer to thirty, I began drawing on my academic background in anatomy, physiology, and physical therapy to really look at the impact that the chronic stress and excessive training were having on my body. After some reflection, I found that my behaviors weren't very consistent with my priorities of physical and psychological resilience, and an overall high quality of life. I continued introspecting and slowly shifting my behaviors and values elsewhere in my life too. Around 2009, as I began to develop this seasonal model, I also began an incremental but significant overhaul of my life. I pivoted away from chronic summer. It wasn't structured in exactly the same way that I organize it here, but the shift was comparable.

Addressing my exercise addiction, I started training less often, moderating my training intensity when I did exercise, and taking more recovery time in between training sessions. I focused more on strength- and power-building movements, and didn't thrash myself so hard or so often with intense conditioning work. This allowed my chronically under-recovered body more time to recover and heal. At the same time, I adopted a Paleo-type diet, and started noticing new subtle and intuitive seasonal urgings around food, like more sugar cravings in the summertime (which match the seasonal availability of fresh fruit), and a yearning for hearty stews, meaty soups, roasts, and root vegetables come wintertime. My larger social disconnections also became apparent, like the lack of meaningful intimacy and vulnerability in my first marriage. I started paying more attention to personal growth and the value of deeper relationships, gradually extricating myself from summer-type, shallower intimacy by becoming more vulnerable with closer anchor connections (as described in chapter 6).

In other words, I was getting out of chronic summer and pivoting to fall.

No matter your starting point when you pick up this book—whether you're in the throes of stress addiction or you still feel pretty good for the moment, yet sense something isn't quite right or believe you can feel even better—chronic summer living has likely left you feeling overstimulated, fatigued, beat down, and a bit unmoored. Our chronic summer civilization has left us, in one way or another, with circadian rhythm dysregulation, dietary imbalances, dysfunctional movement patterns, and a lack of meaningful social connection and self-awareness. This means that we all need an extended period of rest and restoration before we can fully embrace truly seasonal living. Before we can live in a harmonious and coordinated fashion with the seasons of the year, we must normalize, heal, and rebalance our topsy-turvy lives. To offset the damage we've incurred from chronic summer, we must embark on a period of extensive, comprehensive healing—something I refer to as the pivot to fall, followed by a therapeutic winter. I call it a pivot because it's a directional change from our chronic summer's focus on expansion, on consumption, on accumulation.

Chronic summer-style living has depleted us so extensively that, to use a financial analogy, we've all overdrafted our bank accounts. We've overspent our emotional energy, our waking hours, our physical health, our mental bandwidth. To get ourselves out of the red, we need a period of restoration, where we build up our psychological and physiological "savings." The pivot to fall and its deepening into winter is a strategic recuperative strategy—a necessary first step before we can operate on a healthy, sustainable "budget," where our lifestyle incomes and expenditures are roughly balanced. And this means that we can't make partial, compartmentalized changes. If you've racked up some credit card debt, you'll be able to dig yourself out of debt faster if you stop overspending on entertainment or vacations or clothing. But it's only when you address your financial health in holistic terms— examining your expenses on housing, food, transportation, and all the rest—that you can achieve financial health and long-term solvency. Similarly, you can't solve your chronic summer woes just by changing your diet or exercise program while you continue your erratic sleep patterns and self-medicate with likes on social media.

Turning Away from Chronic Summer

By now, we're familiar with my model's understanding of fall—a challenging, directional shift away from summer; a moment of deceleration, energetic contraction, simplification, self-examination, and interpersonal reconnection. We're also familiar with my model's version of winter as a prolongation and intensification of this restorative fall mode—a season of introspection, quietude, deeply nourishing and satiating food, and drawing even closer to our important anchor connections. Up until this point, however, we've been thinking of fall and winter as both seasons in time and as ways to shift behavior as we come out of the high sun of summer and embrace the shorter, cooler days of fall and winter. I've discussed oscillating the four keys of health over the four seasons, embracing summer sleep, eating, movement, and connection in summer, fall habits in fall, and so on across the four seasons of the year. But now, I'd like to expand the reach of these concepts, developing them as metaphors, symbols, and even overarching themes where we deliberately turn away from chronic summer in major areas of our lives.

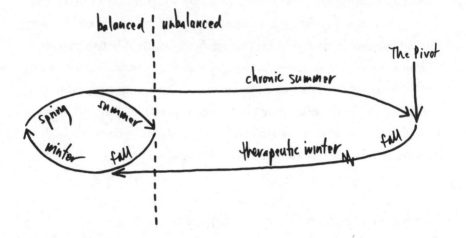

The fall pivot and therapeutic winter each last a minimum of three months (a literal season), and ideally coincide with the actual fall and winter seasons. In optimal circumstances, you'll discover this book in the spring, begin consistently implementing your anchor behaviors in the summer, embark on a pivot to fall in the actual fall, and give yourself three months (or so) of this directional motion before transitioning into the more comprehensive, far-reaching, and deeply restorative habits of a therapeutic winter.

But if you read this book in March or April, I recommend you extend your transition and focus on gradually slowing down. Give yourself a longer period to become mindful of chronic summer as you gradually decelerate and establish the various lifestyle anchors in your life. You don't need to dive headfirst into the fall contraction right away, though you certainly could. If you instead happen to pick this book up in August or September, right as the seasons transition from summer to fall, and feel motivated to begin the pivot right away, do so, but understand that you might experience some attitudinal and behavioral mismatches and it might take a bit longer to fully feel fall's deceleration. Embrace the transition with a spirit of openness and flexibility, and remember that there is no rush. There's no time limit or ideal time frame for this transition; you have many years to let this cyclical approach seep into all the corners of your life. It's okay if you don't make all of the sweeping changes right away. This is *your* journey.

Though not impossible, it's harder to begin the pivot in the warmer seasons because it's a bit unnatural to embrace winter's spirit of contraction in the dog days of summer. Summer's longer days make it tough to relax into a winter restorative mode. And let's face it: it's hard to skip the summertime barbecues, fireworks, long hikes, and social gatherings in favor of staying home, sleeping more, and doing more reconnecting with yourself and those closest to you. Instead of fighting the natural, expansive seasonal urges to go do and see and feel and learn, gradually nudge yourself, and possibly your family, in the general direction of establishing solid anchor behaviors and eating more nutrient-dense whole foods, instead of trying to apply mismatched fall and winter principles in your spring and summer. Once again, it's okay to slow it down. Once you've dialed in your rebalanced lifestyle habits in the literal fall and winter seasons, they are much easier to extend into the warmer months. It's much easier to prolong your contracted social world and general restorative attitude into the spring and summer, and to continue connecting deeply with place and self and others during these months, than it is to start these big contractions during this time.

Here's a guiding principle: coordinate all four keys of symbolic fall and winter with the literal seasons as quickly as is practical for you. And give yourself six months minimum (two seasons' worth) of transition and extended healing once you have. This half-year period of healing is a minimum duration, and given that most of us are extricating ourselves from multiyear or multidecade habits—all of the cultural norms, expectations, conveniences, and habituated pleasures of chronic summer—it might be much longer before we're physically and mentally ready to return to spring-type behaviors. And as we've already seen thus far, the pivot to fall is the hardest shift, as it entails a big directional change away from an exciting adrenaline- and dopamine-fueled summer. Once you've made that directional shift and move from fall to winter, the process will start to feel natural, intuitive, healing, and energizing because you are restoring what chronic summer has depleted.

In past chapters, we've considered each of my models' four-fold variables—sleep, nutrition, movement, and connection—in relative isolation from one another. But we can only make a *lifestyle* pivot to fall and therapeutic winter if we address these variables simultaneously, just as I did over the last decade. As you read this chapter, resist the urge to dismiss any isolated recommendations I offer because you've already tried them or you heard that they weren't really that important. You might have tried blocking out blue light at night, for example, or experimented with a Paleo diet, or tried reconnecting with your spouse in a more meaningful way. You might be interested in ancestral health and may have even incorporated some of the elements of this book into your life. You might have taken on a Whole30 program, or even lived a Paleo lifestyle for an extended period of time, perhaps seeing remarkable shifts in body composition, insulin sensitivity, energy levels, mood, and the reduction of various inflammatory conditions. But while you likely have experimented with different lifestyle variables in isolation, you haven't undertaken the comprehensive fall pivot and therapeutic winter in its totality, approaching sleep, diet, movement, and connection in a concentrated and integrated fashion. You haven't approached seasonal healing in a synchronized way. Well, now's the time.

As I argue in this chapter, one of the causes of our frayed nerves, exhausted bodies, and lonely hearts is that we haven't coordinated these different factors. We've overleveraged summer so badly that we *all* need a period of holistic, comprehensive renewal to get ourselves back on track. Doesn't a pivot to a cooler, slower autumn, and then an extended winter of healing just sound soothing, if perhaps unfamiliar? Yeah, I thought so. Our civilization's destructive chronic summer has bred such imbalance and disease; the solution is a fall pivot and therapeutic winter. Take your foot off the gas, let the engine come down from redline, cool, and simply idle for a while.

Falling into (Better) Sleep

Many people tend to overthink sleep by analyzing, planning, and structuring it, instead of focusing on removing the roadblocks that prevent it from naturally unfolding. A move to fall sleep patterns does precisely that, creating space for our body to achieve the rest, restoration, and recuperation we so deeply need every night.

To prepare your body for sleep each evening, provide environmental cues that allow it to feel relaxed and safe. For several hours prior to sleep, avoid intellectually or emotionally stimulating or stressful movies, books, and other media. If you read an evocative novel or watch a psychological thriller on Netflix, you'll generate emotional arousal and perhaps a stress response that can make it much harder to settle into sleep. In these presleep hours, avoid frustrating or potentially triggering activities, like checking work email or assembling IKEA furniture. Those things will still be waiting for you in the morning. Avoid intense exercise within a couple of hours of bedtime as well. If your schedule dictates that you must exercise in the evening, decrease the intensity dramatically so that you don't generate a stress response that blunts the secretion of melatonin that is required for deep, restorative sleep.

If you must do your exercise in the evening, restorative yoga is better than an intense spin class. If you have a partner with whom you co-sleep, avoid emotionally intense conversations right before bed, as they're very likely to trigger stress and impair sleep. An argument before bed will likely derail ideal sleep.

Avoid caffeine, nicotine, and alcohol at night. Many people use alcohol to decompress, especially if they've had a difficult or stressful day. But there's a stimulating effect of alcohol, too, which is why if you have several drinks prior to bedtime, you'll often wake up or toss and turn midway through the night.[1] For optimal sleep, stop drinking three or four hours before bedtime so you have time to clear it from your system before syncing into that restorative sleep mode. Similarly, caffeine has more of a stimulating, sleep-disrupting impact than you might think. If you have trouble sleeping and you regularly consume caffeine, you have to at least consider its possible contribution to your sleep woes. If you have trouble confining your caffeine consumption to the morning, perform the following experiment: go a week when you drink no caffeinated afternoon beverages and see how your sleep fares. You might think caffeine doesn't have any effect on your sleep because you can drink a cup of coffee and go straight to bed. But that simply indicates that you're exhausted enough to achieve sleep despite chemical stimulation. You might be surprised by what a difference this simple modification can make in your sleep.

To create an environment conducive for restorative sleep, try to eliminate all light and noise pollution from your bedroom. As we discussed in chapter 2, this means avoiding screens, or at the very least acquiring blue light–blocking glasses if you absolutely must be on your computer or phone two or three hours before bed. There are several computer programs and apps, like f.lux and Night Shift, that help filter out those problematic blue wavelengths. If there's any light streaming through your windows, hang blackout curtains or blinds to completely block it, so that your room is dark like a cave. If you are traveling or total darkness at home is not possible for some reason, wear an eye mask to bed. To avoid the abrupt and stressful experience of waking to an auditory alarm (the word *alarm* itself indicates a problem!), I instead recommend a light alarm: a dimmable light bulb that you can program to slowly brighten up your room in the morning, helping you to wake up by mimicking a natural sunrise. Start your day with light! Also consider Himalayan salt lamps that give off a soft, warm glow in the bedroom. Because they match the setting sun's warm color hues, they are especially useful in the evening hours, and I find mine very calming. To reduce the impact of noise pollution, use an analog white noise machine in your room, or download a white noise app (always remembering to put your phone into airplane mode if it's in your room at night).

Make your sleep environment simpler and more relaxing. Clean up your bedroom to make it less visually cluttered; whether it's your preferred style or not, consider a minimalist decor for your sleep space. Think of your bed itself as a place for sleep, sex, and intimate conversation, but not eating, reading, playing on your phone, or watching TV. While avoiding stressful conversation with your partner is key, physical intimacy (with a partner or with yourself) is a great way to create the hormonal climate that helps you relax into a restorative sleep state. Adjust the thermostat for ideal sleep temperatures—around 65°F, or 18°C—and consider a few deep-breathing exercises or minutes of meditation in this cool, dimly lit, relaxing space. Aren't you getting drowsy just reading about this?

A great, final way to achieve better sleep is to create a nighttime ritual. Read a book, snuggle with your kids or companion animal, take a warm bath with Epsom salts and relaxing essential oils like lavender, or have a cup of herbal tea. Keep a notepad next to your bed and if during these relaxing moments you come up with a creative idea or item for your to-do list, write it down. You'll off-load the responsibility to remember it, which allows your brain to relax more completely.

As you read my recommendations for sleep, check in with yourself. Are there any ideas I mentioned that you immediately resist? Go back and reread the above paragraphs, jotting down one or two recommendations to which you feel most resistant—you're either arguing about its validity or dismissing it as particularly useless. These are the places where I want you to start your pivot to a fall sleep pattern. Lean into the places you resist the most, like putting away your fast-paced novel or giving up your 3:00 p.m. cappuccino. What we most strongly emotionally resist is often what will benefit us the most. This principle applies to our other key behaviors too. Notice the things you resist, and instead of reflexively casting them aside, I challenge you to embrace them. I used to absolutely detest yoga, and I've more recently found it to be transformative, but that discovery could only happen once I leaned into the uncomfortable, awkward space. I suspect you'll discover something really helpful once you use the indicator of internal resistance as your guide toward your most impactful shifts.

Becoming a Fall Foodie

Transitioning to fall nutrition might be the most straightforward lifestyle change you'll make during this comprehensive pivot. Because whether you've been immersed in a healthy nutritional paradigm for years or are just beginning to think critically about your diet, the general movement is the same. Fall food selection represents a deliberate resistance to the overwhelming pull of summer's cravings. It's a more moderate nutritional position. Fall's diet is sane and balanced—something that prepares your body to embark on seasonal oscillation for a lifetime.

In its broadest outlines, a movement toward fall eating involves consuming local and seasonal foods and anchoring them around a naturally raised or naturally fed meat, seafood, or egg protein source. Supplement these offerings with liberal amounts of nutrient-healthy fat sources like avocados, nuts, seeds, and grass-fed butter. In a broad sense, the really moderate diet I described in *It Starts with Food* is very much a fall-type diet. You can consult that book, any of the Whole30 resources, or simply return to chapter 3 of this book to orient yourself to fall eating staples and approximate portion sizes.

When prioritizing healthy, nutrient-dense fall staples, you'll naturally eat fewer nutrient-poor and inflammatory foods. Remember that this lifestyle pivot will ultimately serve as a foundation for lifelong nutrition, so focus on what you are prioritizing, not what you're excluding. The Whole30 program's elimination of all added sugars, artificial sweeteners, grains, legumes, dairy products, and alcohol is wonderful and certainly a powerful and healthy way to eat. But it's also a short-term experiment, not an optimal long-term diet. Think of the fall pivot as a gentler, more extended transition period of developing an integrated wellness lifestyle that's flexible and achievable in your life. If you've completed a Whole30 program and you've found its principles energizing, that's wonderful. Take the lessons you learned about your own food sensitivities, satiety signals, and energy levels, and carry them forward as principles, but not rigid rules. Don't be afraid of veering "off-plan," enjoying a sweet dessert treat or an alcoholic beverage on occasion. There's room for occasional deviations because your fall pivot represents a broad directional shift in your journey, not a tight-rope to walk.

To nudge yourself out of habitually consuming high-carbohydrate, high-sugar summer offerings, you might consider a check-in that I do with my son. When he was around age four or five, we started having conversations at the dinner table about how he felt after eating his meal. If he asks for a sweet treat, I cue him to pause, take a few deep breaths, and ask his body whether it's really hungry for dessert. "Look," I'll usually say to him, "the priority here is the nutrient-dense meat and vegetables. If you've eaten all those meat and vegetables and you feel pretty good about things and you want a little bit of a treat, you can have that. But do you really want that right now?"

To my amazement and delight, he'll often decline dessert. And like most of us, that boy loves dessert. "I thought I wanted dessert after dinner," he'll say, "but I realized I'm already full and I don't really want to eat anything else." Alternatively, he'll say, "I feel good and I don't need dessert," or "I don't need extra sugar." At six years old, he's developed an awareness about his own nourishment and satiety, and he continues to hone his self-awareness of his cravings. If we perform this brief check-in, we can all develop such an awareness, whether we're six or sixty-six. When we're deeply nourished and sated with complete proteins, healthy fats, and dietary fiber, we gravitate less to refined carbohydrates and sugar. This isn't a panacea for your sugar cravings (since those are also exacerbated by chronic stress), but it might bump you out of a mindless, lifelong habit of eating dessert after most meals.

Perform this check-in with yourself, not just after dinner but following each meal. Are you craving ice cream, doughnuts, cookies? Ask yourself the following: "If I had a plate of panfried salmon and steamed cauliflower right now, would I want to eat it?" If that sounds appetizing, you are still hungry and should eat more nourishing food. But if you don't want that nutritious meal and instead just want the ice cream, then you're experiencing a sugar craving. That distinction is important when making the transition to fall. People often eat to satiety, especially in the evening, and then out of habit and driven by stress hormones—and the omnipresence of high-calorie, nutrient-poor summer offerings in our environments—reach for a sugary dessert. Sometimes such habits are long-standing, dating back to childhood when parents rewarded us with sugar-laden treats. Once habituated to summer's easy sugar, we self-medicate or self-soothe with sugary (or at least carbohydrate-dense) foods, like candy, French fries, pasta, bread, ice cream, and pastries. Remember, refined carbohydrate gets rapidly converted to blood sugar, so the pleasurable response to pastries is partly driven by the low-nutrient carbohydrate; it's not just the sugar that drives us. Slow down. The pivot to fall requires us to pause, reflect, and consider what our bodies truly need.

Building in the opportunity to develop more self-awareness is quite powerful at the beginning of the day too. Often, out of habit or rush, people skimp on breakfast. It's time to break that habit. At the end of breakfast each morning, ask yourself, "How do I feel? Do I feel like I'm well nourished? Do I feel like I have enough energy now to go out and start my day and power me through to lunch?" If you pause and reflect on these questions, you might discover that you haven't consumed a satiating breakfast. If you only had a banana, a muffin, and coffee for your first meal, you might find that this isn't adequate. (You *will* find that out around 11:00 a.m. when you're ravenous or brain-fogged.) Revisit the protein leverage hypothesis I described in chapter 3 and consider eating a few panfried eggs or sausage (or leftovers from last night's dinner!) to power you through until lunch, stabilizing your blood sugar levels and keeping your mind clear.

A check-in with ourselves helps us curb unnecessary, problematic overconsumption (of sugar and refined carbohydrate) and also address inadequate consumption (of complete protein and healthy fats). But as is the case with everything in the pivot, the most important aspect of fall-style nutrition involves pausing, reflecting, and taking stock. This isn't a dietary experiment in the tradition of a short-term cleanse or a "ten days to flat abs" gimmick. You are instead creating a foundation of dietary wholeness to serve you for the rest of your life, and that starts by leaving behind the old habits that haven't served you well while creating a "new normal" for your better, brighter future.

Autumnal Movement

It's relatively easy to accelerate the transition to sleep. Starting today, you can take a magnesium glycinate supplement before bed and hang blackout curtains in your bedroom, and you'll start to notice positive changes. Likewise, after a month or two of autumnal-style eating, you'll also begin to see positive effects in your life. Exercise is different. Because it involves a structural stressor, we must ease into it more gradually. Getting injured exercising is pretty ironic, don't you think?

This approach needs to be personalized, and largely based on your individual fitness level, before pivoting to fall. In chapters 4 and 6, I described the importance of engaging in functional, strength-based movement patterns like squatting, deadlifting, ascending stairs or steep hills, rock climbing, and picking things up and ferrying them either in your arms, on your back, or in your hands. If you've integrated these movements into your lifestyle for a few months, then you can advance deeper into your personalized pivot. But if you've been relatively sedentary, or performed no strength training at all, you must develop this movement "anchor" before supplementing with the other hallmark fall movements. Please perform the anchor behavior of functional strength training described in chapter 6 for at least a month or two before you add any additional conditioning work. Go slow and easy, remembering that movement and exercise should represent mild bodily stressors that you gradually adapt to, making you stronger and more resilient over time. I'd feel like I failed to provide responsible, helpful guidance if you ended up getting hurt or even further beat up by life's stressors as a result of starting my recommended movement plan.

In general, the pivot to fall movement represents an amplification of the anchor movements. During your pivot, do a lot of low-intensity, high-frequency movement, like walking, stair climbing, and riding your bike to the grocery store instead of driving. To cultivate a spirit of autumnal movement, start to gradually blur the lines between physically active and fully stationary aspects of your life, deliberately and proactively choosing to move and engage more of your body when you can. For example, instead of sitting still on your therapist's couch, ask if you can walk and talk instead, or take some conference calls as you're casually walking instead of stapled to your office chair. When you feel ready, begin integrating higher-intensity activities into your routine. Gravitate away from the long-duration summer activities of hiking, swimming at the lake, playing golf, and gardening and toward higher-intensity movements like hill sprints, intervals on your bike, or rowing (on a river or on a machine).

Generally, your movement during fall's pivot should mark a midpoint between the extremes of low-intensity, long-duration summer activity and the short-duration, maximal intensity of winter. Do fifteen to sixty minutes of beach volleyball, tennis, or pickup basketball. Or train for a five- or ten-kilometer race, start rock climbing, take up Brazilian jujitsu, or sign up for aerobics classes. Diversifying the nature of your workouts is also central to the fall pivot. If you've primarily emphasized a winter-type strength-training regimen such as power lifting or bodybuilding, then you've already built robust connective, muscle, and skeletal tissues. It's now time to supplement with some moderate-intensity, moderate-duration activities to build your cardiovascular endurance. On the other hand, if you've been engaging in chronic summer cardio, introduce some strength training, reducing your total training time and increasing the intensity. In fact, if you're a die-hard CrossFit, Orange Theory, or Insanity participant, or religiously attend the local pseudo-military sergeant's "boot camp" classes in the afternoons, you'll likely work out less during the pivot (just like I did as I tapered down from my excessive reliance on training to manage my psychological stress).

Remember, if we're using an intense exercise regimen to blunt our feelings or to self-medicate, we're off kilter. People commonly develop addictions to intense exercise like hard running, CrossFit, and triathlons, but not to tai chi, hiking, swimming in a relaxed fashion around a lake, and gentle yoga. The first group provokes a stress response, and the second doesn't. Notice that. The kind of exercise I'm advising in the pivot, and eventually for every season, should not negatively affect your psychological state if you skip it.

When I initially began working with consulting clients who struggled with compulsive exercise, I started hearing about their increased irritability and anxiety as we dismantled their destructive training programs. "Isn't this healing work supposed to make them healthier and happier?" my clients' partners and family would often ask. "He's turning into a total jerk and picking fights with me all the time." I realized eventually that their real addiction was to the stress response that intense exercise elicited. My clients were unconsciously addressing their withdrawal from intense exercise—itself a self-medication—through creating interpersonal stress with those closest to them. In other words, they were swapping physiological, structural stress for interpersonal stress—all the same to the body. We do this in all sorts of ways, swapping compulsive scrolling for video gaming, reading and intellectualizing in place of experiencing our difficult feelings.

We avoid and self-medicate in so many different ways, and just like exercise, some of the behaviors look "healthy" on their face, but peel back a layer, and you'll notice that the reason you're doing that specific thing is anything but healthy. Sure, it's probably better to exercise compulsively than to use drugs, but the commonality is the lack of healthy, effective coping skills for unhealed pain and buried trauma. If this resonates with you, I highly recommend digging up some books by Peter Levine, Bessel van der Kolk, Alan Fogel, and Gabor Maté.[2]

Initially, you might experience withdrawal symptoms when it comes to cutting back on exercise (or compulsive socializing or media consumption); you might become cranky when you can't reach for your phone right before bed or finish the day with a big bowl of sugary ice cream. Whenever we try to extricate ourselves from an addictive pattern, we're liable to experience anything from anxiety to irritability, short-term sleep disruptions, negative moods, and a *lot* of resistance to the change. But remember: compulsive exercise is detrimental to your body, and ultimately a sign that you are in the throes of chronic summer stress. The healthy solution to anxiety or depression is not more stress from excessive exercise, though moderate exercise can be a powerful tool. The extrication process might prove psychologically or physically challenging *in the short term*. But you can rest assured that you are making a deeply healing choice as your body adjusts to a more nourishing baseline that can sustain you into a vibrant and robust old age.

Fall-Focused Connections

Whether it's exercise, nutrition, or sleep, so much of the fall pivot involves decelerating from summer's frenzied, topsy-turvy pace. Connection follows the same pattern. Cultivating fall-style connectivity begins with slowing down and reconnecting with ourselves, whether that takes the form of mindfulness meditation, introspection, psychotherapy, or journaling. Sift through the fairly superficial social connections of summer and (re)establish a more profound connection with *you*. As in other areas, the pivot to fall should represent an opening—a cracking of the door. Your goal is just to feel more and to look more directly at larger questions about yourself, your connections, and your larger place and purpose in life. You likely won't answer such questions after several months or even several years. This is a lifelong process, and your pivot to fall's deeper connections is the critical first step. If you don't eventually leave chronic summer behind, you won't have much of an opportunity to explore some of these bigger, deeper topics, and your long-term sense of peace and belonging will suffer.

Make some room for yourself by double-checking on your social engagements. Just as you ask yourself whether you really need dessert, ask yourself whether you really want to attend happy hour every Friday night with your colleagues, or if you really want to host a birthday party for everyone in your daughter's class next month, or if you need book club *and* your weekly basketball league games. Declining some of those social opportunities allows you more time to reconnect with yourself and even your closest friends and family. Another way to socially decelerate is to start recognizing sources of gratitude and recording them in a journal. I used to roll my eyes when I heard people talk about such journals, dismissing them as soft, fluffy, even contrived and self-indulgent. But I don't see it that way anymore. Gratitude journaling is a simple, effective mechanism to notice and connect to a deep sensation of appreciation and gratitude—both hallmark emotions of fall. Of course, you don't have to journal to express gratitude (it simply helps you to notice the things you might be grateful for); you can simply express gratitude as you feel it, to other people, to yourself, to a higher power or to mother earth if that fits your belief system.

In the context of your fall pivot, take some time for other self-care activities dedicated to your personal restoration. Once we start to slow down and notice our needs, a series of helpful self-care activities will often come into focus. They might include the stereotypical bubble bath and glass of wine, rising ten minutes earlier in the morning to meditate or read, or getting a massage every few weeks. These activities need not be expensive nor time intensive. For me, the most important of such activities is meditation. Meditation is the ultimate self-care practice, and a powerful way to be more present and grounded. It's therefore optimal to start during the pivot. I recommend Eckhart Tolle's profound book *The Power of Now* and Dan Harris's *Meditation for Fidgety Skeptics* as starting points. The apps Headspace and Insight Timer are both excellent meditation tools too.

Pivoting to fall also involves connecting or reconnecting to place, people, and purpose. Whether literally or metaphorically, we've spent our summers preoccupied, busy, and traveling—maybe working our butts off on the job or distracting ourselves with Netflix binges. In the spirit of autumnal deceleration and reconnection, think about spending more time settling in at home, decluttering your surroundings and possibly even revamping the decor while you're at it. Reconnection to place might also involve returning to your family roots, to your hometown. As I've observed after two decades of living in America, Thanksgiving is one of the most emotionally powerful holidays. It's the archetypal autumn celebration that honors familial rootedness. Seek that emotional tone throughout your metaphorical fall.

Whether we return home or not, this pivot means reinvesting in and prioritizing our anchor connections. For many of us, these close connections are parents, siblings, children, aunts, uncles, and cousins. For those without such close familial relationships, our anchor connections might be our closest friends or other members of our "chosen family," such as committed romantic partners. These are the deep, intimate, profound relationships that are stable over time and resilient through difficulties. As I've discussed, reconnecting with our anchors or establishing new ones can be awkward and even discouraging because we make ourselves vulnerable to the rejection of others. But fall's directional shift from numerous, more superficial connections to fewer, higher quality ones requires that we lean into the discomfort. That is a move that will take time, energy, and courage.

Begin this reconnective process by checking in on the quality of your relationships. Ask yourself: In what ways are my relationships deep and meaningful? In what ways are they superficial or emotionally distant? How can I bring some of these people closer? Could an acquaintance of mine become a closer friend? Could I connect with my dad in a more profound way? Maybe you could invite your basketball friends to have dinner with you and your family, instead of leaving promptly after your weekly games. Reconnection involves exploring these topics and following up with deliberate and proactive action.

Our chronic summer society encourages superficial and mostly *fun* modes of connection, so be prepared for people to express a little confusion or discomfort when you open up to them or invite them closer. Part of this pivot is learning how to part with your defenses, frustrations, or past hurts and to speak with more openness and vulnerability to others. "We haven't talked much these past few years," you might say to a faded anchor connection. "We ended things with a fight, and I'm ready to put that behind us and reconnect."

Also remember that the fall pivot is a moderate, transitional step. We're not engaging in summer partying, but we're also not only having friends over for an intimate fireside chat in the deep of winter, discussing our existential dilemmas and most profound insecurities. Instead we're deliberately moving toward reconnection in a healthy, experimental fashion. This shift takes time and practice, and fall is the perfect transitional time.

As I discussed in chapter 5, a reconnection to purpose, place, and self are integral parts of this process. The fall pivot provides a great opportunity to check in and reassess the direction of your life, considering whether you are on the right track in your career, friendships, marriage, and even finances. So much of chronic summer society hinges on consumption, and an almost insatiable desire for acquisition, a constant yearning for more. Part of reconnecting to purpose is checking in with yourself, possibly with a close friend or loved one, to help you explore profound questions. Ask yourself: Do I have enough? This is a particularly potent question to ask after doing some gratitude journaling and noting all that you *do* have. Give this some careful thought and consideration, because society's default assumption is that we never have enough. Even if you have a gratifying job, pay all of your bills, and want for nothing, you'll still likely feel the need for more. More money. More recognition at work. More toys. More square footage in your house. More retirement savings. That's the mantra of chronic summer: more, more, more. Consider prayer, meditation, introspection, and journaling as important strategies for questioning our society's default mode of endless acquisition and for identifying your truest desires.

One of the challenges of being in a perpetual summer mode is that we never acquire true knowledge of ourselves, either. Our extrication from the outward focus and consumption of chronic summer includes self-examination, gleaning valuable self-knowledge through inward-looking, quiet, and sometimes solitary experiences. Summer's consumptive mode is necessarily future oriented, urging you to work harder so you can acquire more things, like a bigger house, an exotic vacation, and an elite education for your kids. Mindfulness, by contrast, entails clearly seeing and experiencing what is happening *now*.

The "enoughness" and adequacy of fall often involves being profoundly present. And who knows: your innermost longings and true life purpose might arise spontaneously as you focus on the moment, exploring what you want out of life and whether your current actions match your values.

Take parenting, for example. Parenting might constitute a big chunk of your life purpose. Or, on closer reflection, you might feel that intensive parenting has displaced some greater purpose you have. It's easy to lose ourselves in the parental roles of provider, protector, teacher, nurturer, and chauffeur. There's great beauty in sacrificing your quality of life, time, or energy in the service of your kids; the disconnect happens when parents make these sacrifices out of guilt and social expectation rather than a deep calling. Strike a balance between honoring your values as a parent and honoring what's important to you as a person. You'll be setting a great example for your children by showing them how you take care of yourself and find balance among life's many competing demands.

It's essential to recalibrate this balance throughout our lives because chronic summer overstimulation can numb our deeper yearnings for purpose and meaning. That might even be one of the reasons that we seek out the numbing stimulation—to drown out the unaddressed, gnawing recognition that there is something bigger out there for us. Pivoting to fall provides an opportunity to embrace a more philosophical and introspective mode. This may sound idyllic or romanticized, but often the revelations that arise from these slower, quieter activities are, in fact, deeply unsettling, discouraging, and disorienting, leading us to question some of the fundamental premises about the way we view the world, our personal values, our relationships, spirituality, or the ultimate nature of consciousness. The fall pivot might also be a time of grief and sadness, of the deeper recognition of past losses, leaving you feeling more disoriented than you did in summer. This is one of fall's central challenges and paradoxes: we are more deeply connected to ourselves, our anchor connections, and a sense of place and purpose during this season, yet we often simultaneously feel solemn, discouraged, and might feel a downturn in our mood. It's a paradox we feel keenly at first, as we withdraw from the numbing stimulation of excessive summer.

However uncomfortable or unfamiliar these feelings are, experiencing more of them is a positive sign. As we notice the grief, sadness, and loneliness that we've drowned out in our chronic summer frenzy, we can explore the source of these feelings, and begin addressing them. Maybe we need to explore a childhood trauma in therapy or address a spiritual yearning we have through meditation or prayer. Or perhaps we deeply desire a committed intimate partnership that we don't currently have and need to make some shifts to make room for.

Sometimes this process allows us to push beyond our long-held beliefs and automatic assumptions, and to connect with our more profound inner yearnings. For most of my twenties and thirties, for example, I identified as a hard-line atheist, believing there was no deity or supernatural reality of any sort. But following the introspection and self-evaluation I did during my incremental fall pivot and extended therapeutic winter, that perspective has begun to soften somewhat. I've moved away from a strident position of knowing what I believe to a more flexible space where I'm open to a variety of different spiritual possibilities. I don't really know what I believe, and that's okay. Just broaching those questions has made me more open, compassionate, and self-aware, and has been deeply rewarding and meaningful. Spirituality is one of many ways we cultivate meaning and purpose, and as I've explored this previously unknown dimension of myself, I've experienced enhanced meaning, and that has fueled the trademark fall feelings of gratitude, abundance, and generosity. This whole cluster of profound and interrelated experiences wouldn't have been possible without my deliberate slowing down and peering within as part of my personal pivot to fall.

That's part of the beauty of fall. It's a transitional period, allowing us to make way for the emotional intensity and presence of winter. Then, once spring comes around again, we can experience more outward-directed energy, intensity, and zest—feelings we haven't had much of lately because of our chronic, exhausting summer. Grief, sadness, discomfort, and recognizing things that you need to let go of are typical of fall. Fall is a time of stripping away, of lightening one's psychological and emotional load, and this letting-go process can invoke sadness that we are unaccustomed to feeling (given how much time and effort we spend avoiding discomfort in our collective chronic summer). But fall also catalyzes self-discovery, an enhanced feeling of purpose and contribution, and even the wonder and awe that can arise from mindful meditation or a spiritual practice. Lean into all of those feelings, as they in turn enable the beautiful renaissance of spring and our reemergence as strong, fertile, capable people. As powerful as a fall pivot can be, three months of moderate fall won't undo the consequences of years or even decades of chronic summer. That's why, following our pivot out of that unnaturally long paradigm, we must embark on an even more therapeutic and restorative phase of metaphorical winter—the *true* antidote to chronic summer. Winter is a powerful medicine for our summertime ills.

Winter Heals

As a season of profound recovery, therapeutic winter is grounded in restfulness and sleep. You can think of winter sleep as a recovery period from an illness, literal or metaphorical (or both). Sometimes, when getting over a bad flu or cold, you might sleep for fourteen hours straight, or ten hours a day for five consecutive days. Our therapeutic winter also contains extended periods of sleep, all designed to correct for your prolonged period of pathogenic chronic summer. Experiment with dimming your lights as early as 8:00 or 9:00 p.m. and, if possible, arise naturally with the sun. Don't mistake this extra sleep for lack of productivity or laziness. On the contrary, winter sleep is deeply healing—and necessary.

Therapeutic winter's nutritional staples include meat (including the fattier cuts), preserved foods, and root vegetables like carrots, beets, parsnips, and winter (hard) squashes. Winter is a great time to embark on short-term trials of low-carb/ketogenic and time-restricted eating patterns. With the consumption of high-fat, low-carbohydrate foods your body will naturally shift from burning mostly carbohydrates to relying on more stable fat and ketone sources to fuel it and your overall recovery process. As you know from past chapters, I recommend doing all your eating during the daylight hours. In the wintertime—real or therapeutic—we have fewer daylight hours, resulting in a shortened "feeding window" to consume food, allowing our body to spend less time digesting and more time healing. For optimal restoration, consume your largest meal in the morning within an hour of waking/sunrise, a smaller lunch, and a spare pre-sunset dinner. Not giving in to the after-dinner cravings will be made easier by dimming the lights (thus not sending the "be alert" signals that can cause sugar cravings) and heading to bed earlier. You don't need to exert willpower to not snack if you're asleep! For those of you not habituated to eating breakfast, you'll probably find it easier to eat in the morning if you ate dinner at 5:00 or 6:00 p.m. and didn't snack at all after dinner.

When it comes to movement, think of therapeutic winter as your rest period or (relative) off-season. This is a time to give chronic over-use injuries, like that nagging plantar fasciitis, patellar tendonitis, or lingering shoulder ache, an opportunity to heal. Expending less energy and pushing less hard enables such physiological recovery. Your anchor movement of functional strength training should remain intact, and if you feel energetic and motivated, feel free to engage in the winter-style movements I've described in this book like short bursts of intense movement or interval training. But here's my therapeutic winter rule: your total time spent engaging in continuous high-intensity movement is ten minutes. That means that when you're doing intervals, say, on a one-to-one work:rest ratio, your total time in activity cannot exceed twenty minutes. What I'm getting at here is that the total "dose" of stress is very small; that neither moderate strength training nor very short, high-intensity training induces a large hormonal stress response; that avoiding more stress is a critical feature of a healing winter.

Therapeutic winter similarly opens you to psycho-emotional healing. Because we've removed the excessive and superficial summer relationships, winter's connection to self and our closest others becomes more intense (in a really good way). Winter is a time to deepen any introspection and self-awareness activities you've embarked on during your fall pivot. During therapeutic winter, you'll be home and perhaps alone more, simply relaxing, reading, journaling, napping, daydreaming, and meditating. Let yourself get bored. Let your mind wander. Give yourself permission to *not* do things. If you didn't start therapy or a daily meditation practice during the fall pivot, do so now. Talk about what you discover with a few close anchor connections, and go deep. As the pendulum swings the farthest away from the superficiality of summer, winter is a time for terrifying intimacy and profound vulnerability. Strongly consider going on a social media blackout during this season. I know one person who gave up his smartphone entirely for his therapeutic winter. I admire that kind of commitment to one's own healing process. Admittedly, I struggle with engaging "just a little bit" with social media, and I foresee more offline blackouts in my future as I continue to expand my own healing into more corners of my mind and life.

Keep in mind that, especially when contrasted with the spring-summer continuum of which we've grown long accustomed, winter's general vibe can sometimes feel a bit solemn. Therapeutic winter entails a natural downturn in mood, when feelings of loss and the awareness of mortality can arise. Winter is the time when the trees *look* barren or even lifeless, but it's also the time when they are storing up resources to rebound into rapid growth and expansion in the spring. As a summer society, we aggressively avoid such difficult emotions, regarding them as "bad" or even pathological. When we pivot to fall and then therapeutic winter, we thus experience these submerged feelings that have often gone unresolved for years or decades. Don't fear natural human experiences of grief, loss, mourning, and sadness. To the extent you can, embrace them. (Not to minimize truly pathological depressive conditions that must be addressed professionally; do not hesitate to seek out professional help if needed.) Winter—seasonal and therapeutic—is a normal time to process these cyclical emotions of loss, loneliness, and sadness, leaving you less burdened when you resurface in spring, lighter and clearer.

Establishing or finding a long-lost connection to purpose often comes out of deep winter's introspection. That purpose sometimes has a spiritual component, an interpersonal or relational component, or a societal dimension. It virtually always involves something larger than ourselves. Most of the time, our most peaceful, meaningful, gratifying life experiences occur in relation to people, whether that person is us, our families, or our larger communities. Whatever your purpose in life might be, don't rush therapeutic winter's restoration and don't skip past the opportunity to be present to your feelings, thoughts, dreams, and disappointments as you struggle to find your purpose and path. You're not going to sort this out in a few weeks or even a few years, but each gleaming winter provides more opportunities to learn and deepen your connection to purpose. This evolution of self goes on forever, which I find both maddening and magical.

For some people, as I've mentioned, a season of therapeutic winter might be fairly brief, perhaps only a few months. Younger readers in particular might need less of a therapeutic winter, as they handle stress better from a physiological perspective and haven't had as many years of exposure to chronic summer stimulation. They're simply not so badly beaten down. For others, especially people with systemic inflammation, mental health struggles, or metabolic dysregulation, their therapeutic winter might last several *years*. Mine did, and I revived this principle for a second go-around as part of my postdivorce healing process. I'm not saying that your multiyear therapeutic winter should be a period of full-blown ketosis, minimal movement, and social isolation. It simply means that you'll concentrate the range of activity and lifestyle variation during this period toward the winter end of the seasonal continuum, even in the actual spring and summer seasons. The fall pivot and therapeutic winter entail more of a dominant mood, feeling, or orientation, instead of a fixed set of objective behaviors. You can have a healing, wintery *mind-set* even if it's hot and sunny outside.

If, for example, you are a night-shift worker or travel extensively, your body experiences perpetual circadian rhythm disruption, making fall sleep a challenge. Speaking plainly, this is a sub-optimal situation. But that doesn't mean you can't still do a fall pivot. Instead, it underscores the importance of offsetting an imperfect situation with even greater consistency across the *other* lifestyle keys, making great dietary choices and achieving consistency with movement and social behaviors. Perhaps you have an orthopedic injury like a meniscal tear in your knee or some chronic inflammatory condition that doesn't permit intense exercise or skeletally loaded strength training. That's all right too. During your pivot, you can work toward partially loaded (scaled) body-weight movements, or even stand up and down out of a chair a few times. Do what you can and build from there. This is a very flexible system that you can start using no matter where you currently are.

Maybe your schedule is chaotic, you're experiencing financial difficulties, or even grappling with mental illness. You can modify my prescriptions accordingly, working around certain parameters and customizing others. It might take you several years. Some readers might have dedicated years to eating healthy, developed a strong sense of self-knowledge and self-efficacy, and have a supportive close-knit group of family and friends, but might have changed jobs, relocated their families, embarked on new career paths, had a child, or returned to school. These external circumstances also pose challenges, none of which are insurmountable.

I've had hundreds of consulting clients over the years tell me that they couldn't possibly curtail their intensive exercise routines. "It's good for me," they say. "It's camaraderie at the gym. It's social connection. It's stress relief. It helps me sleep better. It manages my weight!" How could I possibly deny them something that has so many obvious benefits? It's a fair question, but it also requires that we examine the underlying motivations, which always end up being more important that what the tangible behaviors are. In these cases, these clients were often rationalizing and defending their addiction to intense and excessive exercise, mounting resistance to a more moderate regimen of fall movement. As anyone who has ever dealt with addicts understands, they are masters of justifying the addiction and denying that there is a real problem. I can say that; it takes one to know one.

Some of my clients have pushed back on my food recommendations, saying that they can't fully get on board with my food plan because the organic, seasonal, sustainably raised food I suggest is elitist, unrealistic, or too expensive. Others protest that they *need* a steady drip of all-day caffeine to keep themselves awake during work; or that they can't part with their cell phones at night because the work taskmaster expects them to be available twenty-four hours a day. There are many challenges that people might have with these changes, some of which are fully valid. We all must pay our bills, and if you absolutely must do overnight shift work to do so, then there's no way around that. Sometimes, however, people will say my dietary plan is too expensive, but nonetheless spend $400 a month to lease a high-end car and $150 for cable television. Affording the optimal food in this case is not a financial limitation, but not a priority relative to other consumer items. It's a statement about personal values. There's no judgment inherent in that; only *you* can determine what's most important to you. Oftentimes, resistance to changes masquerades as a pragmatic limitation. That resistance often really covers up a fear of failure, discomfort with the unfamiliar, fear of social rejection or judgment in being unconventional, or feeling alone and unsupported by your family, friends, or partner. If you're pushing back against some of my recommendations, check in with yourself and ask what the "but what if _____" concern is. I bet it's there somewhere. Sometimes, simply identifying what the fear is helps you to move through it.

But whether you are internally resistant or openly enthusiastic, think of the fall pivot and therapeutic winter as a series of self-directed principles and concepts, not pass/fail propositions and rigid rules, that, taken together, trend toward deceleration, restoration, contraction, and reconnection. The more you embrace these principles and the more broadly you apply them to your life, the smoother and more gratifying of a transition, and future life, you'll ultimately lead.

Once I got past some of my own internal resistances, I greeted fall with relief. I fell into it like a child falls into the comforting arms of a parent. Chronic summer living often felt like I was speeding—recklessly—on the freeway. Sometimes the feeling was momentarily exhilarating, but it was also scary and uncomfortable, as I thought about aggressively slamming on the brakes, swerving, or losing control and careening off into the ditch. The safest and best way to adapt in such circumstances is to simply take your foot off the gas, flick your turn signal, and deliberately move to a slower lane. That first moment of deceleration is immediately calming and reduces your stress response. But notice, you're not screeching to a full stop on the freeway, and you are still in the car on a journey. This figurative deceleration creates an opportunity to inhale deeply and recognize you are shifting in a safer, more positive direction. Like slowing down to a safer, less reckless speed on the freeway, moving into fall gives you more control, safety, room to breathe, time to think, and, ultimately, peace of mind.

Living the Pivot

Do you remember Kim from chapter 1? She was the woman in a familiar rut who bathed in blue light as she tried to fall asleep, engaged in unhealthy movement patterns, and managed only a subpar marriage and so-so relationship with her kids. I have some great news about Kim. I introduced her to the concept of anchors, and she spent a few weeks establishing important dietary, sleep, movement, and social foundations in her life. With those foundational anchors in place, Kim then embarked on the pivot I described in this chapter. She became really consistent in avoiding blue light in the evenings, and instead reads a (print) book of poetry she keeps on her nightstand. She bought a light alarm, allowing her to wake up more naturally and in step with the natural light. She sets it for fifteen minutes before she needs to wake up, so she can take some quiet time to wake up gradually and enjoy a few pages of poetry as she eases into the day.

Once she's up and rolling, her first priority is locating an anchor of complete protein for the family breakfast. Starting the day with protein has given her more energy and a more stable mood. She also purchased a monthly box of produce, commonly referred to as community sup-ported agriculture (CSA), and now eats an array of seasonal fruits and vegetables. It's taken some work and occasionally some research. Kim has found herself with unfamiliar produce on several occasions and had to go online to learn how to cook turnips, rutabaga, and acorn squash, but she's enjoyed the adventure of cooking and eating new foods. With this concentration on local produce and dietary proteins, her household consumption of refined grains and dairy has decreased substantially.

Kim's work schedule is still demanding, but after she ditched her high-intensity workouts and instead focused on movement anchors, she's become much more at ease and happy. She met a few girlfriends at the gym and decided to host them every other weekend for an informal brunch. Nothing fancy—she simply decided to take a risk and draw people with similar experiences and lifestyles closer to her. Her desire for closer, meaningful connection also extends to her husband. Kim and Mark's marriage wasn't in crisis, but they'd been disconnected for a while. After a few conversations, they decided to enter couples' therapy in a proactive attempt to communicate better and connect more deeply. Though they found it a bit awkward communicating before a third party at first, their communication started to improve, and this extended to their physical intimacy as well, and they were both grateful for the experience. Kim and Mark still have their own interests, and they allow each other space to pursue them. But when they do connect, they have more fun—like they did during their marriage's early days.

Paying more attention to each other led Kim and Mark to focus more on their kids. They instituted a very unpopular "no devices at the dinner table" rule, and it was a headache at first. But they led by example, not checking their phones as they talked to each other. As they became more present with each other, they were able to engage in more meaningful conversations with their kids about what was going on at school, and with their friends. Soon, the grumbling about the phones subsided.

Kim's reconnection has also extended to herself. Like many mothers, she'd lost touch with herself in the chaos of parenting. To recalibrate her life, she established a daily, fifteen-minute mindfulness meditation practice first thing in the morning. It was a small lifestyle adjustment, just like her morning poetry reading. But both of these activities have made a big difference, as Kim starts her day feeling centered and creatively nourished, and now feels less frayed, anxious, and fragile.

Three months following her fall pivot, Kim and her husband embarked on their more intensive, immersive experience of therapeutic winter. They naturally started winding down even earlier in the evening. They stopped watching television altogether and moved all phones and non-analog devices from the bedroom, choosing instead to illuminate their space with salt lamps and sometimes burning candles. This increased the comfort and intimacy of their room, and also dimmed the light spectrum, helping them achieve a more peaceful, relaxed nighttime mode. Kim and her husband extinguished the candles at 9:00 p.m. consistently and fell asleep shortly thereafter.

After embracing several months of a fall-style moderate diet, Kim's eating patterns gravitated toward even higher-fat, lower-carbohydrate offerings. She made stews, short ribs, and hearty soups in her slow cooker, stocking leftovers in the fridge or freezing them in ziplock baggies, easily accessible for lunches on the go and even filling breakfasts. Her kids initially looked at her funny: "We're going to have meat stew, for breakfast?" But they grew accustomed to the change, and now instead of thinking of cereal, waffles, and orange juice as breakfast food, they have a broader and richer understanding of food in general.

As Kim's mindfulness meditation practice progressed postpivot, her self-knowledge deepened in turn. During her fall pivot, she'd experimented with erecting boundaries, sometimes telling her children that she needed to redirect their energies when they asked for a late night at the amusement park or arcade. But during her more intensive therapeutic winter, she had more profound realizations about the nature of human boundaries themselves. Prior to this journey, for example, she'd believed that creating boundaries was a defensive or aggressive act. Psychotherapy and meditation, however, led her to understand that boundaries serve to more clearly articulate and define the borders of self. Over the span of fifteen years of marriage and parenting, she realized that the boundaries between herself and her family had blurred, leading her to neglect important self-care and lose sight of her life's purpose.

Armed with these realizations, Kim started carving out more time for herself and began maintaining healthier boundaries with her family and her children. Her morning meditation time became fixed and sacred. She also drew her anchor connections even closer. She and Mark committed even more to couples' therapy, exploring profound topics that made them feel close, connected, and intimate (though also more vulnerable and exposed than their fall sessions). The kids started relying less on their phones and exploring more creative pursuits. Kim's daughter expressed an interest in taking art lessons, and Kim began drawing and painting herself, becoming closer with her child in the process.

Overall, Kim is more emotionally stable and present for her kids, her husband, and herself. She hasn't lost copious amounts of weight—in fact, the scale reads the same as it always did—even though her clothes fit her better. Feeling more settled in her life, she's proactively advocated for herself and her own interests, choosing to stay in and connect with people over homemade meals or brunches instead of going out for drinks. She also declined to take her children to the water park one weekend, telling them instead that she needed more family time with them (and more time with herself). She did this lovingly, without aggression, modeling for her kids how to establish healthy boundaries, even when it came to them. Ultimately, for Kim, this six-month period of movement away from chronic summer has given her more rootedness, control, and sense of connection.

———

In many ways, Kim's fall deceleration and embrace of winter restoration is far from revolutionary. Over the course of the twenty-first century in particular, our society has begun to realize it's collectively disconnected, lost, and frayed at the edges. Many studies, for example, have drawn attention to the importance of prioritizing sleep. There's a larger cultural conversation around how sleep is deeply restorative, and integral to one's mood, mental health, cognitive performance, and longevity. People have started to pay more attention to sleep hygiene, wearing blue light–blocking glasses to work on their computers at night, and even avoiding screen time altogether before bed. And that's a step in the right direction.

The importance of healthy, nutritional eating has also broadened throughout our society. When the Whole30 program began crystallizing around 2009, it formed part of a larger movement of popular nutritional awareness, during which people began experimenting with plant-based diets, low-carbohydrate or ketogenic diets, and seasonal, local eating. And while we know junk food is bad, it's also common knowledge that sedentary lifestyles are just as unhealthy. At this point that's as ingrained as knowing that cigarettes are bad for you. Sedentary lifestyles, we've been told in many forms, have profoundly negative effects on our quality of life. We're also aware that conventional aerobic exercise and the type of chronic cardio I describe in this book isn't the best alternative to no movement. In fact, a broad cross-section of North Americans now understand that summer modes of intensive exercise don't create durable bodies that endure into old age. Gyms, personal trainers, and wellness-inclined individuals have begun featuring bodybuilding exercises, step aerobics, and kickboxing, realizing that our long-term structural, metabolic, and mitochondrial health greatly benefit from such activity.

Around 2010 or so, I began noticing a lot more cultural conversation around the value of human connection. Sherry Turkle's *Reclaiming Conversation* and Susan Pinker's *The Village Effect* join other books in addressing our society's disconnection, loneliness, and overstimulation. Many of us have started realizing that even though we have many "friends" on social media, we still feel lonely. Even technology company executives have put limits on their children's screen times, and app developers have created tracking software to give us awareness about how much time we spend on them. Many of us are startled by how addictive our screen-based entertainments and habits are. We now understand that the social isolation and disconnection that social media breeds are huge risk factors for anxiety, depression, and other forms of mental illness, and we actively limit our screen time, downloading tracking apps on our phones to curtail the time we spend mindlessly scrolling our social media feeds.

As someone whose life purpose centers on health and human wellness, I'm inspired by these positive trends in our society. I've personally experienced how such shifts in lifestyle behaviors have profoundly improved my life, and those of my clients. But what I've also noticed is that however beneficial such isolated and piecemeal lifestyle changes can be, they alone don't produce enduring change. In fact, I've observed the opposite, where people discover ketogenic eating, or high-intensity interval training, or engage in social media detoxes, and believe they've found *the answer* to all the problems that ail them. Unfortunately, these positive changes begin to peter out months or years later, after which time people often double down on the same strategy (pursuing keto with even more ferocity and dedication), or try another isolated strategy, considering the previous one a failure. What makes my model unique is that it combines and coordinates these various principles into an integrated and oscillatory pattern. If you pursue the restorative, health-promoting lifestyle behaviors over seasons, in a coordinated fashion, you'll make lasting, lifelong changes.

But in order to experience the cognitive, physiological, and psychological benefits of seasonal living, we must first embark on a period of restoration. So please: whether you've read books on sleep, tried the Paleo diet, or even actively engineered your biological circadian rhythms around morning light and evening blackness for optimal sleep, don't skip this step. After you establish your anchors (see chapter 6), lean into your fall and winter periods in a prolonged, focused, and comprehensive way.

I can personally attest to how indispensable these six months are.

Around 2006 and 2007 I started making changes around my food, and around that same period, I also began moderating my exercise. It was a powerful improvement and I felt better. But it wasn't until I emerged from my therapeutic winter that I really began to feel differently. I embarked on this after my fall pivot, following a period of intense travel, work-related stress, and a divorce. I felt overdrafted and withdrew. I attended fewer social events, dramatically reduced my exercise, slept a great deal, and consumed more fat-rich and hearty foods, naturally curtailing my carbohydrate intake. After decades of a chronic summer, I felt like an injured and sick animal who crawls into a dark hole somewhere to rest and recover.

It was a solemn and hard period, but it wasn't depressing; in fact, it was a period of great clarity, punctuated with moments of joy. Prior to my fall pivot and therapeutic winter, I'd been doing a lot of travel for public speaking. During this period of restoration, I gave myself permission to decline most of these invitations, accepting 10 or 20 percent of those I previously had. Winter's contraction gave me the clarity to understand I needed less travel, and traveling less helped fuel this recovery. Embracing therapeutic winter's spirit of contraction was honoring the deep yearning I had to slow down, nest, and reconnect, especially with my primary anchor connection, myself.

I started introspecting and asking personal values questions like, "What is important to me? What do I care about? How do I want to show up in the world?" Though this time was dedicated to personal growth, as I sought to find my purpose and place, I didn't become a hermit, nor was I completely sedentary. But I did strip back my exercise to the anchors of functional movement and strength training—a few pull-ups and push-ups and moderate-intensity squats—interspersed with walking and light hiking. That was a way for me to maintain basic capacity without increasing stress. I was able to find a much greater

sense of peace, quietude, and restfulness in the solitude of my meditation practice, and in the company of my more intimate relationships
with close anchors. I simply embraced the opposite of chronic summer, leaned into the healing, and emerged with more clarity, enhanced
purpose, and greater energy.

Remember that the joy, reward, and pleasure that therapeutic winter provides is fundamentally different than that of summer and spring.
It brings deep satisfaction, healing, and the promise of a better life. It's
like going to sleep after you've been exhausted for days. You wake up
not feeling spring or summer's sense of exhilaration. Instead you feel
the quiet energy and bountiful restoration that a great night of sleep
provides. I encourage you to embrace a pivot to fall and therapeutic
winter like me and "Kim," approaching your life and wellness in a tar-
geted, comprehensive, and healing manner, enabling you to get out
of chronic summer's debt and embark on sustainable seasonal living.
This period of restoration is worth it. Once this healing is over, you'll
emerge on the other side, ready for spring. You'll have restored previously tapped-out energetic resources, fueling yourself for the psychological, physiological, emotional, creative, and relational expansion
and growth of springtime.

After a prolonged foray into your therapeutic winter, you'll naturally start to feel the telltale markers of spring-style behavior—you'll
start to feel antsy and spontaneously energetic. Look for those trademark feelings of spring: curiosity, excitement, anticipation, optimism.
They often coincide with the literal dawning of seasonal spring. Your
mood will lift, your energy will rise, and suddenly, your interests might
pique when a friend suggests a road trip, or you might have thoughts of
starting jujitsu, rock climbing, or composing music again. The visions,
plans, and dreams that have been hibernating and incubating during
your fall pivot and winter healing may begin to surface, and you might

want to return to school, pick up an old hobby, sport, or activity, or expand your social circle.

Once you detect multiple signs suggesting a personal springtime—like an interest in a new hobby or a strong urge to host a party—you can be sure you are on a positive, healthy springtime trajectory. You'll emerge healed, unburdened with chronic summer's debt, and ready to live a life attuned to the seasonal changes. As we explore in the next chapter, once we've pivoted to fall and emerged from a therapeutic winter, we're ready to embark on a more balanced, seasonal oscillatory pattern, aligning our four health keys of sleep, diet, movement, and connection to the passage of the annual seasons, as well as the seasons of our lives.

CHAPTER EIGHT

Your Life Beyond

Congratulations. You've completed your therapeutic winter. It took you about eighteen months, but you sure feel stronger and more physically capable. No more inflammatory conditions, and fewer achy joints. Your prediabetes is mostly gone, and your doctor tells you to ditch those blood sugar medications. You enjoy stable energy, and that nagging midafternoon energy slump has largely vanished. Mentally and emotionally you feel much clearer, more stable, settled, emotionally resilient, and creative. Because you've slowed down enough to introspect, you've adopted a different mind-set and way of evaluating your life as you've explored more profound questions about your larger purpose. You're finally ready to start living in a balanced oscillatory fashion, in harmony with the changing seasons. Join me now on an imaginary journey, as I give you a taste of what seasonal living will look and feel like.

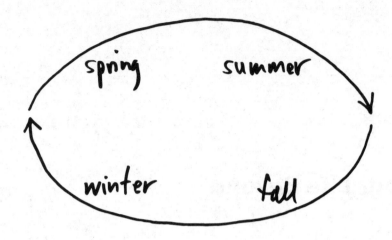

Each spring, you'll emerge from winter's relative slumber feeling like a brighter, lighter, happier, and more energetic version of yourself. Your friends will likely comment on your glowing skin or suggest that you exude or radiate something positive, something they can't quite identify. In the spring of each year, you're inclined to try new things, go new places, and start thinking about a new hobby, relationship, or career possibility. Absent chronic summer stimulation, you embrace these experiences every year, leaning into spring's titillating fun and excitement. Sometimes your spring ideas are harebrained, and you try them out anyway.

If you run a small business, each springtime you can anticipate more energy at the office. You aren't driving to work when it's still dark outside, and the extra sunlight alone gives everyone a little more zest and pep. Each spring you capitalize on this energy surplus and organize an open forum to generate ideas for the coming fiscal year. You consider new business operation approaches and start planning a big sales push or product launch for the upcoming summer. These anticipatory plans are galvanizing for your teams, managers, and general employees alike, and you leverage those positive feelings to create camaraderie in the office.

When it comes to your marriage, you look forward to spring because it's a period of novelty, energy, and playfulness. Linda Carroll's *Love Cycles* textures a cyclical relationship model that dovetails with my seasonal model.[1] As we all know, long-term romantic relationships can feel settled, comfortable, and a little complacent over the course of time. But, to put her ideas in my seasonal, oscillatory idiom, Carroll suggests you take advantage of springtime's telltale trait of novelty to reinvigorate your relationship. This is the time, she says, to interact in a fun and playful way, trying new things or even reverting to some of your relationship's springtime behaviors, from your puppy love or honeymoon phase.

In her book *Mating in Captivity*, psychotherapist Esther Perel describes the oscillatory dynamism and tension between familiarity and novelty in long-term relationships.[2] Spring is your ideal time to have conversations with your partner about expansion, novelty, and growth. And this isn't confined to romantic partners. Each spring I look forward to talking with my son. "Man, we've had a nice, quiet winter," I tell him. "We've been at home a lot. What do you want to do this summer?" And the two of us start planning for climbing camp or summer backpacking and camping trips.

My mother, Debbie, has always been active, healthy, and outdoorsy, planning long backpacking trips with her girlfriends. One spring day, when she was about to turn sixty-five, we were stunned by the manner she'd chosen to mark the milestone: she decided she would hike an 800-mile section of the Pacific Crest Trail, the fabled pathway that runs from Mexico to Canada. Even professionals have difficulty with it, and my mom decided to hike hundreds of miles of it. Alone. Every springtime Mom starts readying herself for the upcoming summer journey.

Each spring, she's excited to embark on the planning phase as she anticipates the next leg of trail she'll cover, the mountaintops she'll scale, and wildlife she'll encounter.

My mom's hike is perfectly in keeping with the spirit of seasonal spring, brimming as it is with opportunity for new experiences and adventures. As someone who lives on her own, on over one hundred acres in British Columbia, Canada, Mom can pay more attention and honor her own intuitions and desires. She cuts her own firewood, plants her own vegetable gardens, and harvests fruit from her own trees. I'm not saying she's a perfect exemplar of seasonal living, but she's someone attuned to the natural rhythms of the earth and helped instill them in me from a young age. It's gratifying to watch her intuitively embody parts of my model, even as I'm a bit terrified to think of her alone on this trail. As my mother clearly demonstrates, springtime's possibilities aren't confined to youth—they are accessible at every age. And neither are the bold, daring, and sometimes dangerous adventures of summer as my mother hikes several hundred miles of the trail each year.

Each summer of your life, you also behave like my mom, throwing yourself headlong into the projects and experiences you charted in spring. During these months you are brave and daring when it comes to meeting new people and embracing new experiences. You travel to a country where you don't speak the language after you implement the harebrained idea you hatched with your business team during your springtime planning session. Sometimes you are up so late at the office, making these project deadlines, that you get home late, and don't get as much sleep. You dedicate the weekends to renovating the house, restoring your vintage car, and progressing on your woodworking projects. That's perfectly in keeping with non-chronic, seasonal summer as a period where you immerse yourself in intensive experiences and career callings. You also allocate large chunks of time to spontaneous experiences with a wide group of people.

For many summers in my twenties, between twenty-five and forty of my friends rode motorcycles from Salt Lake City to Wyoming. Imagine these bikes loaded down with camping gear, and the fun and mischief we would all have camping together in the woods, embracing what I now regard, in hindsight, as summer's expansive mode. Now that I parent a school-age child, I understand that summer is a season when you might heavily invest time and energy into your kids. They aren't at school all day, or busy with their homework and extracurricular activities. During the summer of 2019, when my son was six, I deliberately arranged only part-time childcare—I still wanted to work—because I wanted to embrace a summer style of parenting and all the attention and emotional energy required for being present with a small child. My son and I had a blast going on weekend camping trips, learning how to light a fire, and looking out for bears and other wildlife on the trail.

Each summer, I've seen my mom turn into a bigger, more invigorated version of herself, as she expands the boundaries of her comfort zone, and increases her confidence and life satisfaction from embarking on something challenging and scary. As you can imagine, she's inspired a lot of people. But I'm equally proud of her for not confining the seasonal experience to her summer. Unlike many who hike the trail, she hasn't set aside a calendar year to do the entire thing. At the end of August each year, when summer draws to a close, she looks forward to coming home, reconnecting with her land, and seeing the friends she's missed from being away for several months. That's because she's naturally tapped into fall's spirit of homecoming and yearns for reconnection and deceleration. After literally expanding her world each summer, she equally embraces the joy of fall reconnection, and all the people and activities she's missed during her adventures away.

Having already recalibrated and rebalanced your life during your own fall pivot, your calendar fall each year resembles the gentle life contraction that my mom manifests. You intuitively start slowing down, spending more hours at home, and paying more attention. You restart the meditation practice and journaling practice that got away from you during summer and begin reconnecting with the people you haven't seen all summer because they've been away traveling or busy working. In our hectic world, summer is a time of natural drift and disconnection, while fall is a warm invitation to reconnection. Instead of going to the lake, fair, or amusement park, you spend more time in your living room or harvesting produce from your vegetable garden. As you reconnect to self, place, and others, you start experiencing spontaneous feelings of gratitude and fullness. You also check in with yourself, asking whether you are on track with your life purpose. I know that my mom is doing this work in the fall of 2019, asking herself whether she made the right choice about ending her year's hike a bit early because of early inclement weather in the northern stretch of trail she was on. (Answer: right decision, Mom.)

You also find value in each fall's preemptive and proactive questioning of important parts of your life. Because rarely do you introspect during this time and conclude, "Yes, I am in perfect harmony with the life I'm leading and my connection to purpose." Fall instead is a time to question and mildly course-correct, rather than waiting until it's too late and you experience career burnout, a divorce, a family estrangement, or the fallout from an affair. Many of my friends, sometimes tongue in cheek, perform an annual marriage or relationship "check-in." Fall is the perfect time for such a meeting. "Where are we in the course of this relationship?" they ask their partners. Most of the time, when you slow down long enough to ask yourself the question about whether you are on track, the answer is "Not quite."

As you've also discovered, fall's spirit is retrospective. This is when you assess and evaluate the business plans you conceived in spring, then implemented in summer. How did that big product launch or marketing drive turn out? Do you want to do the same next year, or do you want to modify, or change course more dramatically? Fall isn't the time to dwell on the past—it's a time to learn from it, evaluating it with a spirit of curiosity and openness. During fall's retrospection, you sometimes discover that you've neglected parts of your exercise routine. It's fairly painless, you find, to return to movement after having gone off track for one season. In fact, deciding to get back into regular exercise initially requires some effort, but proves enriching. That wouldn't be so if you'd been off track for years, whether that manifests in no activity or an exercise addiction.

When you engage in cyclical fall's nourishing behaviors, you don't feel the exhilaration of dopamine-driven summer. Instead, you feel healthy pride. Such pride stems from proactively evaluating your relationships and big projects. Sometimes this involves healing an old friendship damaged by some misunderstanding, opening up new channels of communication and intimacy with your romantic partner, or reinvigorating your relationship to self with enhanced journaling and meditating. No matter the particulars, fall feels like the opposite of chronic summer's fatigue, anxiety, depression, and exhaustion, all of which stem from self-medicating with alcohol, processed foods, television binges, and other analgesics. Armed with self-awareness, a sense of peace washes over you each fall, as you course-correct important parts of your life, realizing that these changes have the potential to manifest in a future that can be even richer than your past.

This nourishing fall provides a great foundation for your average annual winter, a time of comfort, quiet, and mild healing. Having resisted the "go go go" impulse of those in thrall to chronic summer around you, you actually look forward to this time, and the deep connection and intimacy with loved ones it entails. You don't feel giddy and happy every winter, but you sure feel rooted and rested. Instead of looking externally for self-validation and self-respect, you practice self-care and feel authentically restored and recharged as you explore interpersonal and intrapersonal connection with your anchors. Each winter you lose yourself in a great book and look forward to playing board games with your kids and parents.

After I left for home for university, my parents contacted me before winter break. "You don't really need anything," they said. "And we don't really need anything. Why don't we just skip Christmas gifts this year?" We skipped them and it was wonderful. No one stressed out about what to buy. It's a tradition I've happily continued my entire adult life. I realize that this is a significant departure from the cultural norm, where Christmas has morphed from a religious celebration to an orgy of consumerism. But summer's spirit of consumption is seasonally mismatched with winter's intrinsic contraction. The more I veered away from the compulsive, mindless shopping component of Black Friday and Christmas, the more peace, quiet satisfaction, and gratitude I felt.

Your family doesn't abandon Christmas or holiday gift-giving like mine did. But after leaning into fall's feelings of generosity and bounty even more over the course of several winters, you tuned into your deeper yearnings and intuitions and decided to scale it back. You realized that our chronic summer civilization, which makes holiday gift-giving obligatory, is out of sync with the spirit of generosity you feel when congregated with your family over the winter holiday season.

During those winter celebrations, as you enjoy a cup of good cheer and reminisce with your family, you experience a different dimension of generosity. In that space of acceptance and belonging, your family is naturally unselfish and spontaneously generous. And that sense of profound connection and generosity you feel is so fundamentally different from consumerist-oriented Christmas that one year you decided to venture into the community with that same spirit, exercising generosity with those less fortunate by serving in winter soup kitchens and volunteering at winter clothes drives. Since it involves entering the community, such an act might immediately strike you as a spring- or summertime behavior. But if you slow down during fall, and notice your adequacy and abundance, winter can become a season when this can manifest as charity toward others. If Thanksgiving is the hallmark expression of autumnal gratitude, generosity and service to others is its natural expression in the winter that follows.

As you spend years and decades living in sync with your natural biological rhythms, each of these seasonal iterations becomes progressively more harmonic and intuitive. Each seasonal change presents you with the opportunity to reassess, recalibrate, change course, and continually evolve. And this ultimately makes you stronger. This is partly because the seasonal model leverages the power of the "novice effect": an accelerated adaption to a new stimulus. The novice effect is typically discussed in exercise circles, when people embark on training for a marathon or a new weight-lifting regimen and experience rapid improvement, adaptation, and progress. Thanks to the "novice effect," the new athletes' bodies are highly adaptable to the initial stimulus (in this case, new bodily movements). The farther they venture into that same set of practices, however, the less significant the adaptation becomes.

When living in a continuously oscillating seasonal mode, we can harness the power of the novice effect, creating opportunities for rapid and accelerated adaptations to new foods, movement styles, and so forth, every season. Every single winter that you embrace higher-protein and fat-rich foods, veering toward a lower-carbohydrate or ketogenic diet, the more rapidly you'll experience improvements in your insulin sensitivity, and the more efficient your body will be at using fat as a fuel source. When pivoting to the consumption of a broad range of local fruits and vegetables each summer, you ingest a large array of phytonutrients and minerals that serve as powerful antioxidants or agents of bodily detoxification. The metabolic flexibility you've acquired in the seasonal model allows you to quickly adapt to these new minerals, helping you to offset such things as solar radiation in the summertime. Seasonal living allows us to continually prompt ongoing adaptations to new stimuli across the course of a lifetime, rendering our bodies and psyches more flexible and durable.

And if achieving the novice effect and balancing the four keys sounds intimidating or hard to achieve, remember that all my seasonal behaviors are mutually reinforcing. Once you start making positive changes in one area or lifestyle key, the more this catalyzes positive changes across the others. It's been gratifying to see this play out in the Whole30 community. As online message boards amply attest, when people embark on a one-month Whole30 plan and aggressively change their nutritional eating patterns, many experience larger improvements in their lives. Their anxiety suddenly clears, their OCD symptoms improve, they sleep much better, and are even inspired to leave unhealthy relationships or initiate larger career changes. Upon the conclusion of the program, I've heard the following phrase more often than I can count: "I'm strangely happy." What they're feeling is a physiologically normal healthy state. They just haven't felt it in so long that it strikes them as weird or disconcerting.

Scientific research further substantiates this general tendency, demonstrating how the adoption of certain parts of the seasonal model can help reinforce larger improvements across your life. For example, research has shown that increased gut permeability, a condition that can be caused or exacerbated by a diet high in refined vegetable oils, sugar, and refined carbohydrates, allows a chemical called endotoxin, which comes from gut bacteria, into the bloodstream.[3] This endotoxin, other researchers found, increased the response of a part of the brain called the amygdala to socially menacing representations.[4] Given that the amygdala is responsible for rapid self-protective responses, this means that people with poor physical health—in this case, a leaky gut—are more likely to be threatened in social situations. If someone's facial expression, for example, isn't particularly soft, welcoming, and friendly, the amygdala of someone with gut permeability is more likely to interpret this in a highly negative way, reacting in a protective and distancing manner. That in turn means that such individuals may be more sensitive to social stressors, like fights and arguments, and have a harder time drawing close and being receptive to others.

This paper suggests that poor physical health begets social isolation. But crossover can happen in either positive or negative ways. While negative factors mutually reinforce one another, so do positive ones, as shown among many people who self-experiment with Whole30. So don't be intimidated by what seems like a lot of moving parts in my model. Once you start leaning into healthier nutrition, sleep hygiene, or movement, you'll find that other elements of the model naturally sync into place.

The Seasons of Our Lives

In chapter 7, I asked you to think about the fall pivot and therapeutic winter as a mind-set and attitude. The same applies for the seasons of our lives, but in a grander, more macro scale. Just as the days, months, and seasons of our lives oscillate, so, too, do the general tenor and orientation of our life seasons. Each of us experiences a youthful springtime of our lives, when, on balance, our activities are more exploratory and anticipatory. We then progress to our summer, fall, and winter life phases, each of which also entails a general seasonal mood or mode, even as we oscillate with the calendar seasons in the way I've described throughout this book.

At forty years old, I'm in the early fall period of my life, evaluating and contracting my general behaviors in a deliberate and intensive way. I still experience seasonal spring each year, when I consume fresh spring greens from my garden, begin to rock climb, and make summer plans with my friends and son. But, in keeping with my life season of fall, I undertake these seasonal springtime activities in a retrospective, evaluative, gratitude-based autumnal manner. This general fall tenor of my life feels intuitively right. The more I embrace a larger fall mindset, the happier, more in sync, and more harmonious my experience of life. That's because, over the years and decades, we experience our greatest happiness and fulfillment when coordinating the phases of our lives to the rhythms and oscillations of the seasons.

But unlike the development of anchors, the pivot to fall, and the therapeutic winter, it's impossible to be prescriptive, specific, and detailed when describing the general direction or orientation of multiple decades of an individual's life. The archetypes of each life season I describe below necessarily reflect my personal experiences, my work with clients, and my research on the topic. Some of these will resonate with you more than others. I'd therefore ask you to embrace the general seasonal principles I elucidate. The specific examples of seasonal behaviors I describe are less important than the general moods, dispositions, and overarching characteristics of the life seasons themselves.

Notice, too, the way in which the seasons build on one another in a seamless and successive fashion. When we embrace the novelty of spring and momentarily lose ourselves in a chaotic summer of career growth, productivity, creativity, or parenting, we are then prepared to undertake a profound and meaningful metaphorical pivot to fall. This, in turn, gives us the most settled, peaceful, and meaningful life winter possible, as we consider our legacy to our families, communities, and larger world. Embracing such macro seasonal change gives us an opportunity to live the best, most fulfilling versions of our lives. If we can fully experience each of our life stages in their entirety, we won't experience arrested development and other hardships (like the midlife crisis), and instead greet each phase of our lives with harmony and peace.

Spring

In the springtime of our lives, a time period that roughly spans birth, infancy, adolescence, and young adulthood (zero to twenty-five years old), we engage in many activities associated with the planning and early growth phase of actual spring. During this time, we learn about the world—through formal, informal, and social education from those around us—find our place, and discover who we are. Think of springtime as that period of anticipation and preparation for the summer of our lives—a phase of novelty, exploration, expansion, and stimulation. The seeds we plant in the life garden of our young adulthood often come to fruition in our middle, later adulthood. Make the most of it: study abroad in college, backpack across Europe, switch majors multiple times, quit a job you hate and seek out something else. This sort of experimentation and exploration represents normal, healthy springtime behavior.

Too often we rush young people through this exploratory phase. Acting out of fear, we urge them to focus prematurely and embrace summer's productivity. I should know. I went to university at seventeen, had my master's by twenty-two, and then looked up one day in exasperation and said, "Wait, I just go to work now for forty years? That's the plan now?" In retrospect, I should have taken a year off to travel, play collegiate volleyball, and enjoy diverse experiences instead of excessively focusing on academia and marriage. Both curtailed the exploration phase of my life, artificially accelerating my life's spring season.

Spring is a phase of intellectual and emotional exploration, during which we explore different romantic and sexual partners. I'm not suggesting that youth and young adulthood are phases of sexual promiscuity, but it is biologically and developmentally normal to exhibit a desire to explore ourselves sexually during this period. For this reason, I tend to discourage people from marrying in their early twenties. You're still in a phase of exploration, expansion, and novelty seeking, rendering marriage a premature intensity of commitment.

When we rush or abbreviate springtime, it lingers on incomplete. One day, we wake up, thirty-five years old, with kids, a mortgage, two cars, and crushed with responsibility and unease. We feel agitated, wondering, "Did I marry the wrong person? Did I really want kids in the first place? I'm stuck in this career that I don't love but I can't afford to quit doing." We can feel stuck, stagnant, and trapped in the world we've built for ourselves, leading to psychological stress and even mental breakdown. We might have an affair, leave a relationship, or file for divorce, believing that something more stimulating, exciting, new, and fun exists outside the boundaries of our current lives. If you find yourself in your thirties or early forties with a desire to upend a major part of your life—that is, if a seismic undercurrent is seizing you, telling you to do something destructive—perform some introspection. Probing your feelings might reveal that you failed to complete the developmental work of spring. After all, impulsive, destructive choices are spring's hallmark.

If you recognize any latent exploratory, novelty-seeking urges, try to create nondestructive opportunities for exploration and expansion in your life. Recognize that these innate desires represent a yearning for a lost springtime experience and embark on a plan that's methodical and deliberate. Look for opportunities to explore new things. Maybe that means broaching a conversation with your partner about reinvigorating your sex life, prioritizing travel to new countries, or broadening your intellectual horizons with new books, podcasts, or movies. Take an academic or vocational course, start a hobby, or do something you've always longed to do, like learning to play classical guitar. In other words, bring those urges and desires to light and devise a plan to address your unresolved spring to achieve resolution and peace, without upending the life you've built for yourself.

Summer

The summer of our lives, roughly spanning the years twenty-five to fifty, resembles our society's default normal—the day-to-day activities we see most people doing. As the most productive and generative years of your life, summer involves going to work, paying bills, buying a house, opening a business or making a mark in your career, and having kids. Armed with a better understanding of who you are and what you want out of life, you can begin executing the plans and the dreams you conceived during spring. As we've already explored and likely experienced, it can be easy to lose ourselves in work, children, and family relationships during the summer of our lives. These are the decades when we apply the maximum amount of energy, intention, investment, and work to our lives. These decades are externally focused. "I'm thirty years old," someone might say in his early summer. "I'm working hard to get a promotion so I can become an expert in my field, start my own business, and later scale it to a consulting agency so that I can achieve financial independence in retirement." This future and external orientation is perfectly in keeping with a healthy summer life stage.

During these high-energy decades, it's normal to feel tired (just like we do at the end of each literal summer). While that's to be expected at times, we must moderate a bit because we tend to pursue our careers, financial accumulation, consumption, and even parenting to excess. There's a fine line between working hard for a couple of decades and working yourself to death. But if you're feeling or looking really broken down—beyond normal aging—then you need to physiologically realign.

Look at your skin as an early indication. Intact collagen fibers make the skin look healthy and vibrant, and the release of the summer stress hormone cortisol leads to the breakdown of collagen and the premature formation of cellulite and wrinkles. The chronic breakdown of your skin can occur elsewhere in your body, when constant wear and tear places our connective tissue in a chronic state of stress, manifesting in shoulder tendonitis, plantar fasciitis, ligament inflammation, and meniscal tears. Cardiovascular disease, insulin resistance, and other types of autoimmune disease also represent the long-term consequences of chronic stress (along with genetic predispositions and environmental triggers). As we now know, chronic stress is a primary common denominator underlying most lifestyle-related diseases and general "dis-ease." [5] Watch for signs that you're awash in chronic summer cortisol and need to slow down during this hectic life stage.

When it's time to make the life pivot to fall, it can seem hard or even impossible to abandon the frenzy of summer chaos and excess. This isn't a personal failing; we simply haven't built an economic system in which people can start winding down their summer in their forties. In the most generous reading, societal expectation is that, beginning around forty-five or fifty, you begin flirting with contracting your life, and exiting the full-scale frontal assault of summer living. But people can't often meet this societal expectation as the forties decade often coincides with the advancement of our careers, the securing of promotions, and the accumulation of more money and status. Can you think of anyone you know who's actively planning on decompressing and winding down at forty years old? Though it's intimidating to consider in today's economy, beginning to detach ourselves from summer at that age is biologically normal.

I'm not suggesting that once you turn forty you actively think about retirement. But once you hit this decade, you should begin thinking about changing your patterns in a broad sense, anticipating a transition from the whirlwind of summer to the gentle deceleration of fall. We must begin early because summer's spirit of accumulation, spending, and advancement requires a vast infrastructure and assumes a logic that becomes self-perpetuating and difficult to unwind. The earlier we begin preparing to remove our foot from summer's accelerator, the more painless and elegant a transition we'll experience.

Fall

While the fall of our lives roughly spans years fifty to seventy-five, we should begin preparing for it in our forties. In living seasonally, after all, we've chosen to be mindful, alert, and introspective about the trajectory of our lives, rendering this directional life change a lot easier. I experienced my fall pivot at age thirty-five and thirty-six and have been gently leaning into a transition to my larger seasonal-life fall ever since. I'm still in a summer production mode, contributing and working hard, delivering podcasts, conducting interviews, and writing this book, but I'm also gradually planning for the next few decades. Right now, I'm reflecting on how stimulating, challenging, and exciting summer has been, but also looking forward to a fall slowdown. As I now understand, I couldn't appreciate the reconnective and contractive phase of fall had I not undergone an expansive summer phase.

The fall of our lives is analogous to the fall pivot, a difficult directional change from expansion to contraction and deceleration. Once we hit fall, we'll likely find ourselves weary from summer's excess. But we also might find that following summer's expansion, we have a wonderful fall harvest to enjoy. The more present, mindful, and slow we are, the more smoothly, gently, and elegantly we can transition into this fall mode. Upon reflection, we might discover we need to change our spending habits and discard some of our unnecessary toys and indulgences, like the boat, motorcycle, expensive yearly vacation, or big house. Material goods such as these might have entranced us during the younger, more frivolous spring and summer phases of our lives. But if we can start spending time and money more wisely, we won't be as beholden to the consumerist forces urging us to keep working to accumulate more.

Most of us don't need such reminders. Despite the societal pressures to constantly consume, most people spend their money modestly and judiciously, and still struggle to stay financially afloat. Currently we don't inhabit an economic world in which it's easy for people to transition from the hard work in their life summers, even when they spend money responsibly on affordable homes, simple vehicles, and retirement savings. With the exception of those who are independently wealthy, this means that we must really pay attention to how we spend our disposable income, as this represents one variable we can control. This is akin to the night-shift workers and constant travelers I invoked in chapter 7—their suboptimal sleeping habits don't grant them an exemption from a fall pivot. It means that they must pay special attention to the other variables they can control.

When we forgo fall's spirit of taking stock and slowing down, problems can arise. A midlife crisis, for example, something that typically occurs during the fall of our lives, simply represents an unrecognized yearning for a pivot or directional shift to spring without recognizing it as such. At around forty, forty-five, or fifty, often due to an unresolved springtime, we yearn to return to partying, sexual promiscuity, and impulsiveness. The stereotype of the midlife crisis— the guy who gets a young mistress and a convertible Porsche at fifty years old—typifies someone who didn't honor each season's lifestyle variables to their fullest. Instead of recognizing our deep yearning for a directional shift to contraction, we sometimes redouble our efforts to earn and consume more, behaving in erratic and destructive ways. Midlife crisis or not, around this stage of life we see a spike in divorce rates as children leave the nest, as well as mental health problems and severe crises of identity, as people confront their midlife in this youth-obsessed society.

The reason the directional fall pivot is so powerful is that it gives us a sense of meaning, purpose, and interconnectedness, as well as self-knowledge and self-acceptance. Within such a framework, this creates a space for Thanksgiving's spirit of adequacy, abundance, and gratitude. Most marketing and advertising focuses on convincing us we don't have enough, prompting more consumption and accumulation. To begin to recognize gratitude, arising from a sensation of abundance and adequacy, simply embark on some mindful meditation exercises. If you start this practice for ten or fifteen minutes a day, you'll notice unresolved pain and difficult emotions arising from your body, mind, and heart. But I promise you—you'll also come to feel gratitude. It'll likely crop up spontaneously and represent one of the richest, most profound feelings you've ever experienced.

Gratitude allows us to tap into fall's telltale spirit of sharing. In the same way that each Thanksgiving we spontaneously share the abundance of the crops we've harvested, so, too, we share during the fall of our lives. In the throes of summer work and accumulation, it's hard to be generous, but as we tap into fall's gratitude and abundance, it becomes much easier and more natural. We might express generosity with our time, attention, skills, talents, abilities, or finances. In today's social-media-driven attention economy, generosity of presence and attention are increasingly rare. There's such power in deliberately reallocating our time and attention to ourselves in the way that Kim did during her fall pivot and therapeutic winter (see chapter 7).

When it comes to seasonal change, remember: we can avoid the turbulence, upheaval, and trauma of massive change (and midlife crisis) if we reassess our lives in each of their seasons, and make incremental course corrections along the way. The most gentle, natural, biologically normal way to experience our lives is through sloping and seamless seasonal transitions across the arc of our lives.

Winter

For many people, winter is the most difficult season to fathom, because it inevitably raises the specter of death. As a society, we handle death poorly. When my father died of pancreatic cancer, I was fortunate enough to be with him, holding his hand. After he passed, the hospice nurse quickly called someone—the coroner, I believe—and he vanished within an hour. In the early 2000s, when I worked as an inpatient physical therapist in a hospital, I saw others were similarly removed postmortem, magically disappearing after being zipped into bags and wheeled away. We're accustomed to hiding death in our society and we don't process it well, exacerbating our trauma, depression, and grief. I tend to think that our society's morbid fascination with horror movies, psychological thrillers, murder mysteries, and serial killers is because they represent some of the few socially acceptable, non-taboo ways we can acknowledge and engage with death.

Ours is a youth-obsessed civilization, where we dye our hair, subject ourselves to cosmetic surgery, and banish the elderly to retirement homes. We're discouraged from thinking about our own deaths, too, leaving the winter of our lives predictably lonely, sad, depressed, and filled with grief. But while it's easy to think of this season in dark, morbid terms, remember that after winter comes spring with new leaves appearing on the trees, and crocuses, daffodils, and hyacinths cropping up from the ground. While we as individuals might perish (physically or eternally, depending on your religious or spiritual inclinations), our legacy, sense of purpose, generosity, abundance, and prosperity can live on in future generations. That doesn't mean it's easy to grapple with our own demise. In the same way that a sense of loss and grief is normal in each literal winter, it's also normal to experience grief and loss in the winter of our lives. But when we experience meaning, purpose, social interconnectedness, self-knowledge, and self-acceptance, and have a sense of contribution beyond our lifetimes, death loses its menacing, fearful overtones. We might even think about our own mortality as an opportunity.

People with the strongest sense of purpose feel most at peace when they die. My father's cancer diagnosis in his early sixties gave him nineteen months to experience an accelerated life winter. Because he lived with a strong sense of purpose, contribution, and generosity, and due to his belief in the afterlife, he accepted his own mortality. He let go of life gently, and in a way that I found—and continue to find—inspiring and beautiful. His peace allowed my mother, sister, and me to grieve earlier, faster, and more completely, and to achieve a sense of closure and gratitude earlier. We miss him dearly. But in the throes of my own life's summertime when he died, I now recognize a beauty and grace in his passing that at the time I couldn't possibly have appreciated back then.

I'm reluctant to speak too specifically about life's winter phase—not because I don't honor it, but because like many people I lack older mentors or elderly figures experiencing the late fall or early winters of their lives who could impart their wisdom to me. It would be arrogant and hubristic for me at forty years old to tell people how they should live at age seventy. My wish is that every reader arrives at the late fall or early winter of his or her life like my mom: strong and bold enough to embrace new adventures. And when you arrive at the end of your life winter, I hope you're like my dad: feeling good about how you've lived and ready to accept your death. In establishing some of the rhythms, patterns, and behaviors that I discuss in this book, and course-correcting for a prolonged life summer, I'm looking ahead to future decades, hoping that when we arrive at late winter, we can lean into the peace, gratitude, and acceptance that we began cultivating in the fall, exiting the world proud, knowing we contributed something of value. I strongly urge you to start that process in a gradual and incremental fashion now, because it's difficult to accelerate when winter is already upon us. The more we align our values, goals, and beliefs with a larger seasonal oscillation, the better life we'll lead along the way, and the better prepared we'll feel when our life span draws to its inevitable end.

As I described in the Introduction, I grew up in an unusually simple world. My parents were unconventional, and never got caught up in society's consumerism and materialism. That remained true even when we moved from the farm and embraced a more mainstream life in my later childhood. And yet, despite the values my family modeled, I was still allured by chronic summer. My seasonal model, which has been gestating since early childhood, and which began to crystallize over the span of a decade, was refined in the quiet, introspective crucible of my postdivorce years. During this therapeutic winter, when I recovered from an acutely stressful period of prolonged summer, I was able to ponder and introspect. And the outlines of my model began to form. Come spring, the contours of the model took on increased coherence and detail, while in the summer, I embarked on the most intensive phase of articulating the boundaries of seasonal oscillation as I wrote and edited this book. During the upcoming fall and winter, I'm looking forward to slowing down, decompressing, and restoring myself so that come next springtime, when the book is released, I can embrace an exploratory, expansive, and energizing mode for my book tour, as I seek to share the message of seasonal oscillation with the world. Undertaking this process in harmony with seasonal change feels natural and right.

In a more macro sense, having corrected for my prolonged chronic summer with a fall pivot and therapeutic winter, I've begun to enter the larger fall phase of my life, where my larger attitude, orientation, and value system is dedicated to decelerating, rekindling neglected relationships, and behaving with generosity. I've just begun to experience the sublime sensation of gratitude within myself and the sense of abundance in my life. I don't spend every moment feeling profoundly grateful for everything around me and lavishing generosity on my loved ones. But having experienced a taste of that feeling has left me wanting more.

As I can attest, we don't achieve perfect seasonal alignment all at once. I'm now forty years old and not sure what the next phase of my career holds. It's uncomfortable to embark on the deceleration of fall living. Connection to self and others was a late addition to my model and something that I have only more recently come to appreciate, value, and enact in my life. I'm doing a lot of catching up with self-appreciation, self-awareness, self-acceptance, and self-gratitude. In an ideal world, I would have progressively deepened my self-knowledge starting in the adolescence and early adulthood of spring, with the assistance and encouragement of mentors, leaders, peers, friends, and close connections. But without my prolonged chronic summer, perhaps I wouldn't have experienced the deep healing and introspection that allowed me to devise this model and write this book.

I'm certainly a work in progress. Confession: I have four motorcycles. Sure, it's been fun having four motorcycles. One's a dirt bike, one's a vintage bike, one's a fast street bike, and one's a more comfortable bike for cruising around town. Superficially, I can justify why I need four motorcycles, but deep down I know that I'm neither a collector nor a professional, and thus don't need them all. In my pivot to life's fall, I'm trimming down on summer's excess, embracing the custom bike that I personally designed and built, and putting two of my other motorcycles up for sale. Such moves are gradual and incremental, as I recalibrate where I've gone off track and continually reevaluate: Am I on the right course? Does this feel good for me? Do my behaviors align with my values? Am I matching my behaviors to the literal seasons and the seasons of my life? There's a never-ending opportunity for improvement, because you're never going to achieve perfection. But by living seasonally, you will achieve more peace, contentment, health, and wellness.

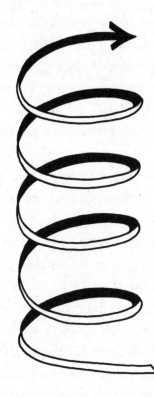

When we align our behaviors and mind-sets with the seasons of the year and the larger stages of our lives, we can achieve harmony with our deepest intuitions and desires for meaning, connection, and contribution. As we oscillate season upon season, year after year, and decade upon decade, we can have the richest, most beautiful and meaningful experiences a human life can have. And that's not because getting more sleep or eating seasonal foods is going to give your life a greater sense of purpose. I've presented the sleep, eat, move, and connect behaviors throughout this book in hopes of removing most of the roadblocks, hindrances, inhibitions, and limitations we routinely create or encounter as we live our lives, so that you can establish your own processes and achieve a healthy buoyancy along life's journey. Once we clear the fog, we create spontaneous opportunities to express our highest potential and live the truest and most beautiful versions of ourselves. This has been a book about pausing and engaging in more disciplined behavior so we can better appreciate and savor life, ultimately achieving optimal health. Because as we've discovered, people can achieve remarkable heights when they are well-rested, well-nourished, physically strong, and socially connected.

As you experience life's oscillations throughout the seasons and years, I hope you will evolve my model, adapt it to your own life, and modify it in different ways, passing along the changes you've found meaningful and gratifying to others. Let this model serve as a launching pad or initial road map in your journey to self-empowerment, self-knowledge, self-expansion, and self-ascension. Use this model to develop the confidence to spontaneously and perpetually adapt my principles, making them work for you practically. My fondest wish is that this book will unlock opportunities to know yourself better and to express yourself more fully, so that your experience of the world is richer, and your deep and satisfying sense of contribution is as large as you want it to be.

ACKNOWLEDGMENTS

The ideas contained in this book have been rolling around inside my head for a long time, and there's a good chance they would never have seen the light of day without the help and encouragement of my dear friend and brilliant colleague, Jamie Scott. He was one of the first to see my initial concepts, and they wouldn't be half as coherent without his insight and research. Mate, I'll be forever grateful. This book absolutely would not have happened without you.

This book also would not have happened without my parents, who taught me to value our connection to the earth and its changing seasons. You planted the seeds for my way of life and my way of thought. Thank you for charting this course for me from the very beginning.

To my son, Atticus, who always inspires to me to live a better life, to be a better person, and to imagine a better world: thank you for being my beautiful beacon in the dark. I love you, sweet boy.

During the long days (and sometimes late nights) of wrangling and writing, my partner, Syanna, was consistently present, patient, insightful, and supportive. Darling, you stuck with me through this entire process, and God knows that wasn't easy. Thank you, thank you, thank you. You're an amazing woman. BT.

I'd like to offer huge thanks to my agent, Lisa Grubka, for your steady hand, patient heart, and guiding influence. You make navigating the publishing world bearable for a simpleton like me, and that's a true feat. Thanks for giving it to me straight and in carefully measured doses. It's been a pleasure to walk through this together. Let's do it again in ten or twenty years.

I'd also like to express gratitude to the entire team at Fletcher & Co., including Christy Fletcher, Melissa Chinchillo, Gráinne Fox, Brenna Raffe, and Elizabeth Resnick. Without your support, this project wouldn't have gone anywhere. Thank you for all your hard and sometimes thankless work.

Without the insight and guidance of my talented and ever-patient editor, Sarah Pelz, this book would still be a hodgepodge of loosely connected ideas. Thank you for seeing the potential in this project from the first day we met, and for helping me weave the complexity into a coherent tapestry instead of a hopelessly knotted ball of yarn. And this book might have gotten written but would never have seen the light of a bookstore without the contributions of the incredible team at Atria, including Lisa Sciambra, Melanie Iglesias-Perez, Dana Trocker, Bianca Salvant, Libby McGuire, and Suzanne Donahue. Thanks to all of you for your contributions.

There are several people who labored intensively on helping me hash out ideas and refine their presentation. A very special thank-you to Seth Schulman, Rachel Gostenhofer, Jamie Scott, and Syanna Wand. Your inputs made this book much, much better.

There are a few friends in my life that I wish I had met many years earlier; Pilar Gerasimo is one of those people. Pilar, you're the most amazing mentor, sister, colleague, friend, podcast cohost, and collaborator that I could imagine. I'm grateful beyond words for your consistent presence in my life.

I often describe myself playfully as an accidental author. At my core, I'm a scientist, a clinician, a thinker, and a teacher, but the opportunity to share my ideas in book format would never have happened without the mountains of work done by the coauthor of my first two books, Melissa Hartwig Urban. Thank you, Melissa, for being my coconspirator and travel partner for all those years. Similarly, I'd likely not be publishing this book without the pivotal influence of Carl Richards. Carl, you gave me a springboard to a bigger and more exciting world. Thank you for all your support and brainstorming. Thanks to Robb Wolf for being an early and generous supporter. I'm here in part because of you.

Ideas need friends too. Thanks to Emily Deans, Andy Deas, and Clif Harski for being friendly supporters of the original concepts that form the backbone of this book.

And to the long list of friends and colleagues who have provided timely words of encouragement, helpful childcare (Julie, Kaleb, and Koda!), resonant sounding boards, and innumerable cups of coffee, thank you.

APPENDIX: SEASONAL EATING

Given the incredible variety of available foods and growing seasons worldwide, it's impossible to provide an accurate, comprehensive seasonal food guide. Instead, I've created a rough guide for the area of the world I'm most familiar with (the northern United States and Canada), and you'll have the opportunity to adapt this to your own locale. Even within the US and Canada, there's an enormous range of locally and regionally available food, so I'm certain that parts of this list will be incorrect for some readers, so think of this as a sample list. If you have no idea where to start when it comes to eating locally and regionally, that's totally okay—you're starting now! Even if you never plant your own garden or raise your own chickens, you can still seek out local farmers' markets and inquire at the local supermarket about which produce items are regional for you.

As I discussed in chapter 6, it's important to get a solid source of complete protein with each meal, and that is best achieved by eating naturally raised/naturally fed animal protein sources such as meat, seafood, and eggs. I have also written about these options and why I recommend them in my first book, *It Starts with Food*. I do not, as a general rule, recommend the consumption of grains, dairy, and legumes.

ANCHOR PROTEIN SOURCES

Grass-fed and organic beef, buffalo, lamb, elk, venison, etc.

Wild-caught and sustainably fished fish and seafood

Pastured, organic eggs

Pasture-raised chicken, turkey, duck, etc.

Pasture-raised pork, wild boar, rabbit, etc.

Processed meats such as bacon, sausage, and deli meat are less
recommended and tend to be harder to find from excellent sources

PRODUCE BY SEASON
(VEGETABLES AND FRUIT)

Spring

Apples	Onions
Arugula	Parsnips
Asparagus	Peas (snap and snow)
Beets	Radicchio
Broccoli	Radishes
Cabbage	Rhubarb
Cauliflower	Scallions
Chives	Shallots
Collard greens	Spinach
Fiddlehead ferns	Sprouts
Kale	Strawberries
Lettuce (all varieties)	Swiss chard
Mushrooms	Turnips
Mustard greens	Watercress

Summer

Apricots

Arugula

Beets

Blackberries

Blueberries

Broccoli

Cabbage

Carrots

Cauliflower

Celery

Cherries

Cucumbers

Currants

Eggplant

Endive

Fennel

Garlic

Green beans

Lettuce (all varieties)

Melons

Mushrooms

Nectarines

Okra

Onions

Peaches

Peppers (sweet and hot)

Plums

Potatoes (new)

Radicchio

Raspberries

Scallions

Sprouts

Summer squash

Sweet corn

Tomatoes

Zucchini

Fall

Apples

Arugula

Beets

Broccoli

Brussels sprouts

Cabbage

Carrots

Cauliflower

Cranberries

Fennel

Garlic

Grapes

Leeks

Lettuce (all varieties)

Mushrooms

Onions

Parsley

Parsnips

Pears

Potatoes

Pumpkins

Quince	Carrots
Radishes	Garlic
Raspberries	Kale
Rutabagas	Leeks
Scallions	Mushrooms
Shallots	Onions
Sprouts	Parsnips
Sweet potatoes	Pears
Turnips	Potatoes
Winter squashes (acorn,	Rutabagas
butternut, buttercup)	Shallots
	Sprouts
Winter	Sweet potatoes
Apples	Turnips
Beets	Winter squashes (acorn,
Cabbage	butternut, buttercup)

You may have noticed that I omitted tropical fruits like mangoes or bananas from this list. That's not to say that you shouldn't eat these foods, but they should play a minor role in your diet during the colder months when the days are shorter. If you choose to consume these foods, either because they grow locally for you or simply because you enjoy them, cluster them primarily in the summer months when high-sugar fruits would be more "expected" by your body. Generally speaking, I'd discourage eating fruit and vegetables that have to be imported from another continent or from thousands of miles of away. One of my favorite markets in Salt Lake City limits their produce to what can be supplied within an overnight drive from the market, and I think that's a great, simple guideline for regional fare. In short, though, don't get hung up on any of these details. Consider this appendix a sample application of a broader principle.

There are also tons of good food options that are less seasonally variable in their availability. These options tend to be less perishable and higher in fat, which makes them ideal choices to supply important dietary fats, especially in the winter months when the variety and supply of carbohydrate-rich plant foods is somewhat diminished and your seasonal shift is naturally toward a higher-fat, lower-carbohydrate diet. As I discuss in *It Starts with Food*, it's very important to choose the highest quality animal products, so if you eat meat or animal fats such as butter or lard, do your best to find a naturally raised/fed source.

Animal fats (preferably from pastured/organic sources)

Butter and ghee (preferably from grass-fed cows)

Coconut oil

Extra-virgin olive oil, avocado oil

Almonds, almond butter

Avocados

Brazil nuts

Cashews

Coconut, coconut milk

Hazelnuts

Macadamia nuts

Olives

Pecans

Pine nuts

Pistachios

Seeds (flax, pumpkin, sesame, sunflower)

Walnuts

NOTES

Introduction

1. For an overview of hunter-gatherers, please see Emma Groeneveld, "Prehistoric Hunter-Gatherer Societies," *Ancient History Encyclopedia* (December 9, 2016), https://www.ancient.eu/article/991/prehistoric-hunter-gatherer-societies/.

2. These dates are approximate. See Graeme Barker, *The Agricultural Revolution in Prehistory: Why did Foragers become Farmers?* (Oxford; New York: Oxford University Press, 2006), 13–29 *et passim* for a history of dating.

3. Leon Kreitzman, "How the 24-hour Society Is Stealing Time from the Night," *Aeon,* November 22, 2016, https://aeon.co/ideas/how-the-24-hour-society-is-stealing-time-from-the-night; "Effects of the Industrial Revolution," *Modern World History* (interactive textbook), accessed September 11, 2019, https://webs.bcp.org/sites/vcleary/ModernWorldHistoryTextbook/IndustrialRevolution/IREffects.html.

4. See, for example, Peter Just, "Time and Leisure in the Elaboration of Culture," *Journal of Anthropological Research* 36, no. 1 (Spring 1980): 105–15.

5. Signe Dean, "Every Single Cell in Your Body Is Controlled by Its Own Circadian Clock," *Science Alert* (October 2, 2015), https://www.sciencealert.com/your-body-has-trillions-of-clocks-in-its-cells; Flávia Dourado, "Discerning the Biological Clock of Single-Celled Organisms," Institute of Advanced Studies of the University of São Paulo, May 27, 2015, http://www.iea.usp.br/en/news/single-celled-organisms.

6. For more on Frankl's philosophy about happiness and purpose, please see Emily

Esfahani Smith, "There's More to Life Than Being Happy," *Atlantic*, January 9, 2013, https://www.theatlantic.com/health/archive/2013/01/theres-more-to-life-than-being-happy/266805/.

7. Thomas Paine, *Thomas Paine: Major Works* (Lulu.com, 2017), 601.

8. Michael Pollan's *In Defense of Food: An Eater's Manifesto* (New York: Penguin Press, 2008) is a great place to start.

9. Maslow later nuanced and clarified his thinking about satisfying lower-order needs and ascending the hierarchy. Please see my discussion below and Saul McLeod, "Maslow's Hierarchy of Needs," *Simple Psychology*, updated 2018, https://www.simplypsychology.org/maslow.html.

Chapter One: Beaten Down by Being Normal

1. "Does Your Body Temperature Change While You Sleep?," *sleep.org* (National Sleep Foundation), accessed September 12, 2019, https://www.sleep.org/articles/does-your-body-temperature-change-while-you-sleep/.

2. Ibid.

3. Ibid.

4. Ibid.

5. Vijay Kumar Sharma and M. K. Chandrashekaran, "Zeitgebers (time cues) for Biological Clocks," *Current Science* 89, no. 7 (October 2005): 1136–46.

6. For the harmful effect of disease, please see "Blue Light Has a Dark Side," *Harvard Health Publishing*, updated August 13, 2018, https://www.health.harvard.edu/staying-healthy/blue-light-has-a-dark-side.

7. Ganda Suthivarakom, "Share a Bed Without Losing Sleep," *New York Times*, March 18, 2019, https://www.nytimes.com/2019/03/18/smarter-living/wirecutter/how-to-share-bed-sleep-partner.html.

8. Ibid.

9. William J. Cromie, "Human Biological Clock Set Back an Hour," *Harvard Gazette*, July 15, 1999, https://news.harvard.edu/gazette/story/1999/07/human-biological-clock-set-back-an-hour/.

10. Sujana Reddy and Sandeep Sharma, "Physiology, Circadian Rhythm," *StatPearls*, updated October 27, 2018, https://www.ncbi.nlm.nih.gov/books/NBK519507/; Willemijntje A. Hoogerwerf, "Role of Clock Genes in Gastrointestinal Motility," *American Journal of Physiology-Gastrointestinal and Liver Physiology* 299, no. 3, September 2010, doi: 10.1152/ajpgi.00147.2010.

11. Paloma Cantero-Gomez, "From Time to Energy Management or How to Learn the Art of Living," *Forbes*, October 24, 2018, https://www.forbes.com/sites/palomacanterogomez/2018/10/24/from-time-to-energy-management-or-how-to-learn-the-art-of-living/#5e3452e97e14.

12. Ibid.
13. Alice G. Walton, "Your Body's Internal Clock and How It Affects Your Over- all Health," *Atlantic*, March 20, 2012, https://www.theatlantic.com/health /archive/2012/03/your-bodys-internal-clock-and-how-it-affects-your-overall -health/254518/; Jonathan Fahey, "How Your Brain Tells Time," *Forbes*, October 15, 2009, https://www.forbes.com/2009/10/14/circadian-rhythm-math-technology -breakthroughs-brain.html#276b8ffe3fa7.
14. Alice G. Walton, "Your Body's Internal Clock and How It Affects Your Overall Health."
15. Ibid.
16. Ibid.
17. "Melatonin and Sleep," National Sleep Foundation, accessed March 27, 2019, https://www.sleepfoundation.org/articles/melatonin-and-sleep.
18. Some call it the "Dracula of hormones": "Melatonin and Sleep."
19. "Melatonin and Sleep," National Sleep Foundation.
20. Kewin Tien Ho Siah, Reuben Kong Min Wong, and Khek Yu Ho, "Melatonin for the Treatment of Irritable Bowel Syndrome," *World Journal of Gastroenterology* 20, no. 10 (March 2014), doi: 10.3748/wjg.v20.i10.2492; Reza Sharafati-Chaleshtori et al., "Melatonin and Human Mitochondrial Diseases," *Journal of Research in Medical Sciences* 22, no. 2 (January 2017), doi: 10.4103/1735-1995.199092; Antonio Carrillo-Vico et al., "A Review of the Multiple Actions of Melatonin on the Immune System," *Endocrine* 27, no. 2 (July 2005): 189–200; Kavita Beri & Sandy Saul Milgraum, "Rhyme and Reason: The Role of Circadian Rhythms in Skin and Its Implications for Physicians," *Future Science* 2, no. 2 (April 2016), https://doi .org/10.4155/fsoa-2016–0007.
21. Thomas A. Wehr, "Melatonin and Seasonal Rhythms," *Journal of Biological Rhythms* 12, no. 6 (December 1997): 518–27, https://doi.org/10.1177/074873049701200605.
22. Michael J. Kuhar, Pastor R. Couceyro, and Philip D. Lambert, "Biosynthesis of Catecholamines," in *Basic Neurochemistry: Molecular, Cellular and Medical Aspects* 6th ed., G.J. Siegel et al., eds. (Philadelphia: Lippincott-Raven, 1999), available from: https://www.ncbi.nlm.nih.gov/books/NBK27988/.

Chapter Two: It Starts with Sleep

1. P. B. Laursen, "Training for Intense Exercise Performance: High-Intensity or High-Volume Training?" *Scandinavian Journal of Medicine & Science in Sports* 20 supplement 2 (October 2010): 1–10, doi: 10.1111/j.1600-0838.2010.01184.x; M. Wewege et al., "The Effects of High-Intensity Interval Training vs. Moderate-Intensity Continuous Training on Body Composition in Overweight and Obese Adults: A Systematic Review and Meta-Analysis," *Obesity Reviews* 18, no. 6 (June 2017): 635–46,

https://doi.org/10.1111/obr.12532; Micah Zuhl and Len Kravitz, "HIIT vs. Continuous Endurance Training: Battle of the Aerobic Titans," accessed September 13, 2019, https://www.unm.edu/~lkravitz/Article%20folder/HIITvsCardio. html.

2. Morgan Manella, "Study: A Third of U.S. Adults Don't Get Enough Sleep," CNN, updated February 18, 2016, https://www.cnn.com/2016/02/18/health/one -third-americans-dont-sleep-enough/index.html.

3. Neil Howe, "America the Sleep-Deprived," *Forbes*, August 18, 2017, https://www.forbes. com/sites/neilhowe/2017/08/18/america-the-sleep-deprived/#38559f0e1a38.

4. Ibid.

5. Gandhi Yetish et al., "Natural Sleep and Its Seasonal Variations in Three Pre-industrial Societies," *Current Biology* 25, no. 21 (November 2015), doi: https://doi .org/10.1016/j.cub.2015.09.046.

6. Ibid.

7. Meg Sullivan, "Our Ancestors Probably Didn't Get 8 Hours a Night, Either," UCLA Newsroom (October 15, 2015), http://newsroom.ucla.edu/releases/our-ances tors-probably-didnt-get-8-hours-a-night-either.

8. Ibid.

9. A conclusion that Richard G. "Bugs" Stevens, professor of medicine at the University of Connecticut, arrived at as well: "We Don't Need More Sleep. We Just Need More Darkness," *Washington Post*, October 27, 2015, https://www.washington post.com/posteverything/wp/2015/10/27/we-dont-need-more-sleep-we-just -need-more-darkness/?noredirect=on.

10. Ibid.

11. See this revealing profile for more: Linda Geddes, "What I Learned by Living without Artificial Light," BBC (April 25, 2018), http://www.bbc.com/future /story/20180424-what-i-learnt-by-living-without-artificial-light.

12. "Why Americans Can't Sleep," Consumer Reports, updated January 14, 2016, https://www.consumerreports.org/sleep/why-americans-cant-sleep/.

13. See the National Optical Astronomy Observatory's (NOAO) figures and recommended illumination thresholds for various indoor spaces: "Recommended Light Levels," accessed September 13, 2019, https://www.noao.edu/education/QLT-kit/ACTIVITY_Documents/Safety/LightLevels_outdoor+indoor.pdf.

14. For all the facts and figures related to Linda Geddes, I relied on Geddes, What I Learned by Living without Artificial Light."

15. Lorenzo Lazzerini Ospri, Glen Prusky, and Samer Hattar, "Mood, the Circadian System, and Melanopsin Retinal Ganglion Cells," *Annual Review of Neuroscience* 40 (July 2017): 539–56, https://doi.org/10.1146/annurev-neuro-072116-031324.

16. Haruna Fukushige et al., "Effects of Tryptophan-Rich Breakfast and Light Exposure During the Daytime on Melatonin Secretion at Night," *Journal of Physiological Anthropology* 33 (November 2014), doi: 10.1186/1880-6805-33-33.

17. T. Kozaki et al., "Light-Induced Melatonin Suppression at Night After Exposure to Different Wavelength Composition of Morning Light," *Neuroscience Letters* 616 (March 2016), doi: 10.1016/j.neulet.2015.12.063.

18. B. S. Alghamdi, "The Neuroprotective Role of Melatonin in Neurological Disorders," *Journal of Neuroscience Research* 96, no. 7 (July 2018): 1136–49, doi: 10.1002/jnr.24220.

19. Y. Li et al., "Melatonin for the Prevention and Treatment of Cancer," *Oncotarget* 8, no. 24 (June 2017), doi: 10.18632/oncotarget.16379.

20. G. J. Elder et al., "The Cortisol Awakening Response—Applications and Implications for Sleep Medicine," *Sleep Medicine Reviews* 18, no. 3 (June 2014): 215–24, doi: 10.1016/j.smrv.2013.05.001.

21. Michelle Dickinson, "Nanogirl Michelle Dickinson: Are Dim Lights Making Us Dimmer?" *NZ Herald*, February 10, 2018, https://www.nzherald.co.nz/lifestyle/news/article.cfm?c_id=6&objectid=11990507.

22. Elie Dolgin, "The Myopia Bboom," *Nature* (March 18, 2015), https://www.nature.com/news/the-myopia-boom-1.17120.

23. R. W. Lam et al., "L-Tryptophan Augmentation of Light Therapy in Patients with Seasonal Affective Disorder," *Canadian Journal of Psychiatry* 42, no. 3 (April 1997): 303–6; Sherri Melrose, "Seasonal Affective Disorder: An Overview of Assessment and Treatment Approaches," *Depression Research and Treatment* (November 2015), doi: 10.1155/2015/178564.

24. J. M. Booker and C. J. Hellekson, "Prevalence of Seasonal Affective Disorder in Alaska," *American Journal of Psychiatry* 149, no. 9 (September 1992): 1176–82; S. Saarijärvi et al., "Seasonal Affective Disorders Among Rural Finns and Lapps," *Acta Psychiatrica Scandinavica* 99, no. 2 (February 1999): 95–101.

25. Kathryn A. Roecklein and Kelly J. Rohan, "Seasonal Affective Disorder," *Psychiatry* (Edgmont) 2, no. 1 (January 2005): 20–26.

26. "Seasonal Affective Disorder (SAD)," Mayo Clinic, accessed September 18, 2019, https://www.mayoclinic.org/diseases-conditions/seasonal-affective-disorder/symptoms-causes/syc-20364651.

27. Alice Park, "Why Sunlight Is So Good For You," *Time*, August 7, 2017, https://time.com/4888327/why-sunlight-is-so-good-for-you/; Christopher M. Jung et al., "Acute Effects of Bright Light Exposure on Cortisol Levels," *Journal of Biological Rhythms* 25, no. 3 (June 2010): 208–16, doi: 10.1177/0748730410368413; H.Y. Tsai et al., "Sunshine-Exposure Variation of Human Striatal Dopamine D(2)/D(3)

Receptor Availability in Healthy Volunteers," *Progress in Neuro-Psychopharmacology & Biological Psychiatry* 35, no. 1 (January 2011): 107–10, doi: 10.1016/j .pnpbp.2010.09.014.

Chapter Three: Food Doesn't Have to Be So Hard

1. Jared Diamond, "The Worst Mistake in the History of the Human Race," *Discover*, 1987: 95–98.
2. M. E. Zaki, F. H. Hussien, and R. Abd El-Shafy El Banna, "Osteoporosis Among Ancient Egyptians," *International Journal of Osteoarchaeology* 19, no. 1 (January–February 2009): 78–89, https://doi.org/10.1002/oa.978; Rebecca Hersher, "Mummified Egyptian Was Just As Sedentary and Carb-Hungry As Modern Men," NPR (July 26, 2016), https://www.npr.org/sections/thetwo-way/2016/07/26/487505112/mummified -egyptian-was-just-as-sedentary-and-carb-hungry-as-modern-men.
3. V. Lobo et al., "Free Radicals, Antioxidants and Functional Foods: Impact on Human Health," *Pharmacognosy Review* 4, no. 8 (2010): 118–26; Megan Ware, "How Can Antioxidants Benefit Our Health?" *Medical News Today*, updated May 29, 2018, https://www.medicalnewstoday.com/articles/301506.php.
4. Please see Dallas Hartwig and Melissa Hartwig, *It Starts with Food* (Las Vegas: Victory Belt Publishing Inc., 2012), 113–16.
5. Aleksandra Crapanzano, "How Eating More of What You Love Can Make You Healthier," *Wall Street Journal*, May 2, 2019, https://www.wsj.com/articles/how -eating-more-of-what-you-love-can-make-you-healthier-11556822538.
6. Ibid.
7. This material is reproduced from my website dallashartwig.com.
8. See, for example, E. A. Martens, S. G. Lemmens, and M. S. Westerterp-Plantenga, "Protein Leverage Affects Energy Intake of High-Protein Diets in Humans," *American Journal of Clinical Nutrition* 97, no. 1 (January 2013): 86–93, doi: 10.3945 /ajcn.112.046540; Stephen J. Simpson and David Raubenheimer, "Tricks of the Trade," *Nature* 508 (April 17, 2014).
9. Alison K. Gosby et al., "Protein Leverage and Energy Intake," *Obesity Reviews* 15, no. 3 (March 2014): 183–91, https://doi.org/10.1111/obr.12131.
10. Alison K. Gosby et al., "Testing Protein Leverage in Lean Humans: A Randomised Controlled Experimental Study," *PLOS One* (October 12, 2011).
11. Ibid.
12. G. A. Hendrie et al., "Greenhouse Gas Emissions and the Australian Diet— Comparing Dietary Recommendations with Average Intakes," *Nutrients* 6, no. 1 (January 2014): 289–303, doi: 10.3390/nu6010289.

13. Shubhroz Gill and Satchidananda Panda, "A Smartphone App Reveals Erratic Diurnal Eating Patterns in Humans that Can Be Modulated for Health Benefits," *Cell Metabolism* 22, no. 5 (November 2015): 789–98, doi: 10.1016/j.cmet.2015.09.005; Amandine Chaix et al., "Time-Restricted Feeding Prevents Obesity and Metabolic Syndrome in Mice Lacking a Circadian Clock," *Cell Metabolism* 29, no. 2 (February 2019), doi: https://doi.org/10.1016/j.cmet.2018.08.004; Satchidananda Panda, *The Circadian Code: Lose Weight, Supercharge Your Energy, and Transform Your Health from Morning to Midnight* (New York: Rodale, 2018).

14. Anahad O'Connor, "When We Eat, or Don't Eat, May Be Critical for Health," *New York Times*, July 24, 2018, https://www.nytimes.com/2018/07/24/well/when-we-eat-or-dont-eat-may-be-critical-for-health.html.

15. Ibid.

16. See, for example, R. J. Jarrett et al., "Diurnal Variation in Oral Glucose Tolerance: Blood Sugar and Plasma Insulin Levels Morning, Afternoon, and Evening," *British Medical Journal* 1 (January 1972): 199–201, doi: 10.1136/bmj.1.5794.199; Eve Van Cauter, Kenneth S. Polonsky, and André J. Scheen, "Roles of Circadian Rhythmicity and Sleep in Human Glucose Regulation," *Endocrine Reviews* 18, no. 5 (October 1997): 716–38, https://doi.org/10.1210/edrv.18.5.0317; Christopher J. Morris et al., "Endogenous Circadian System and Circadian Misalignment Impact Glucose Tolerance Via Separate Mechanisms in Humans," *Proceedings of the National Academy of Sciences of the United States of America* 112, no. 17 (April 2015), doi: 10.1073/pnas.1418955112.

17. Dan Buettner, "Reverse Engineering Longevity," Blue Zones, accessed September 13, 2019, https://www.bluezones.com/2016/11/power-9/.

18. "Social eating connects communities," *University of Oxford* (March 16, 2017), http://www.ox.ac.uk/news/2017-03-16-social-eating-connects-communities#.

19. Shankar Vedantam, "Why Eating the Same Food Increases People's Trust and Cooperation," NPR (February 2, 2017), https://www.npr.org/2017/02/02/512998465/why-eating-the-same-food-increases-peoples-trust-and-cooperation.

20. Michael Pollan estimates 20 percent in a Stanford profile, and 19 percent in an interview with Grist: "What's for Dinner?" *Stanford University*, accessed September 14, 2019, https://news.stanford.edu/news/multi/features/food/eating.html; "An Interview with Foodie Author Michael Pollan," *Grist*, May 31, 2006, https://grist.org/article/roberts7/.

21. Based on data gathered between 2013 and 2016: Jamie Ducharme, "Almost 40% of Americans Eat Fast Food on Any Given Day, Report Says," *Time*, October 3, 2018, https://time.com/5412796/fast-food-americans/.

Notes

22. Leslie Krohn, "Family Dinner Time? Better Leave the Cell Phone Behind," Harris Poll (June 7, 2016), https://theharrispoll.com/family-dinners-have-customarily-held-a-sacred-place-as-part-of-family-life-holidays-and-traditions-but-what-do-they-look-like-to-americans-today-to-better-understand-what-modern-family-di/.

Chapter Four: Moving to the Rhythm

1. Jacqueline Howard, "Americans Devote More than 10 Hours a Day to Screen Time, and Growing," CNN (July 29, 2016), https://www.cnn.com/2016/06/30/health/americans-screen-time-nielsen/index.html.
2. Lindsey Tanner, "Americans Getting More Inactive, Computers Partly to Blame," WGBH (April 23, 2019), https://www.wgbh.org/news/science-and-technology/2019/04/23/americans-getting-more-inactive-computers-partly-to-blame.
3. Susan Scutti, "Yes, Sitting Too Long Can Kill You, Even If You Exercise," CNN, updated September 12, 2017, https://www.cnn.com/2017/09/11/health/sitting-increases-risk-of-death-study/index.html. See also Keith M. Diaz et al., "Patterns of Sedentary Behavior and Mortality in U.S. Middle-Aged and Older Adults: A National Cohort Study," *Annals of Internal Medicine* 167, no. 7 (September 2017): 465–75, doi: 10.7326/M17-0212.
4. Jamie Ducharme, "A Quarter of the World's Adults Don't Get Enough Exercise, Study Says," *Time*, September 5, 2018, http://time.com/5387221/who-physical-inactivity-report/.
5. Gretchen Livingston, "The Way U.S. Teens Spend Their Time Is Changing, But Differences Between Boys and Girls Persist," Pew Research Center (February 20, 2019), https://www.pewresearch.org/fact-tank/2019/02/20/the-way-u-s-teens-spend-their-time-is-changing-but-differences-between-boys-and-girls-persist/.
6. Associated Press, "Kids Today Are Less Fit Than Their Parents Were," *Washington Post*, November 25, 2013, https://www.washingtonpost.com/national/health-science/kids-today-are-less-fit-than-their-parents-were/2013/11/25/8ecb1f0a-515f-11e3-9fe0-fd2ca728e67c_story.html?utm_term=.9c9de67571fc.
7. Jacob Bogage, "Youth Sports Still Struggling With Dropping Participation, High Costs and Bad Coaches, Study Finds," *Washington Post*, October 16, 2018, https://beta.washingtonpost.com/sports/2018/10/16/youth-sports-still-struggling-with-dropping-participation-high-costs-bad-coaches-study-finds/.
8. Associated Press, "Kids Today Are Less Fit Than Their Parents Were."
9. Ibid.
10. "To Grow Up Healthy, Children Need to Sit Less and Play More," World Health Organization (April 24, 2019), https://www.who.int/news-room/detail/24-04-2019-to-grow-up-healthy-children-need-to-sit-less-and-play-more.

11. Katy Bowman, *Movement Matters: Essays on Movement Science, Movement Ecology, and the Nature of Movement* (Washington: Propriometrics Press, 2016).

12. Peter Beech, "Hard Living: What Does Concrete Do to Our Bodies?" *Guardian*, February 28, 2019, https://www.theguardian.com/cities/2019/feb/28/hard-living-what-does-concrete-do-to-our-bodies.

13. Ibid.

14. "Osteoporosis Fast Facts," National Osteoporosis Foundation, accessed May 14, 2019, https://cdn.nof.org/wp-content/uploads/2015/12/Osteoporosis-Fast-Facts.pdf.

15. See Table 2 in James H. O'Keefe et al., "Achieving Hunter-Gatherer Fitness in the 21(st) Century: Back to the Future," *American Journal of Medicine* 123, no. 12 (December 2010): 1082–6, doi: 10.1016/j.amjmed.2010.04.026.

16. Svenia Schnyder and Christoph Handschin, "Skeletal Muscle as an Endocrine Organ: PGC-1 a, myokines and exercise," *Bone* 80 (November 2015): 115–25, doi: 10.1016/j.bone.2015.02.008.

17. Adam Campbell, "The Stupidest Thing People Say about Diet and Exercise," *Men's Health*, September 30, 2015, https://www.menshealth.com/fitness/a19524094/stupidest-thing-people-say-diet-exercise/.

18. "Physical Activity Guidelines for Americans," US Department of Health & Human Services, accessed May 14, 2019, https://www.hhs.gov/fitness/be-active/physical-activity-guidelines-for-americans/index.html.

19. "Physical Activity Guidelines for Americans" (second edition), health.gov, https://health.gov/paguidelines/second-edition/pdf/Physical_Activity_Guidelines_2nd_edition.pdf, 8.

20. Gabriella Boston, "Fitness through the Ages," *Chicago Tribune*, September 4, 2013, https://www.chicagotribune.com/lifestyles/ct-xpm-2013-09-04-sc-health-0904-fitness-aging-20130904-story.html.

21. Talisa Emberts et al., "Exercise Intensity and Energy Expenditure of a Tabata Workout," *Journal of Sports Science & Medicine* 12, no. 3 (September 2013): 612–13.

22. Gretchen Reynolds, "The Best Type of Exercise to Burn Fat," *New York Times*, February 27, 2019, https://www.nytimes.com/2019/02/27/well/move/the-best-type-of-exercise-to-burn-fat.html.

23. Stephen Seiler, "What is Best Practice for Training Intensity and Duration Distribution in Endurance Athletes?" *International Journal of Sports Physiology and Performance* 5 (2010): 276, 282.

24. For more on Dr. Heke, please see the Ancestral Health Society of New Zealand's "Atua to Matua: Maori 'Ecology and the Connection to Health and Physical Activity,'" YouTube video, 45.31, posted January 13, 2016, https://www.youtube.com/watch?v=GjIY0Fka3TY&t=23s.

25. The remainder of this section borrows heavily from my website, dallashartwig.com.

26. Melinda M. Gardner, M. Clare Robertson, and A. John Campbell, "Exercise in Preventing Falls and Fall Related Injuries in Older People: A Review of Randomised Controlled Trials," *British Journal of Sports Medicine* 34, no. 1 (2000): 7–17; Seong-Il Cho and Duk-Hyun An, "Effects of a Fall Prevention Exercise Program on Muscle Strength and Balance of the Old-Old Elderly," *Journal of Physical Therapy Science* 26, no. 11 (November 2014): 1771–74.

27. Tony Rosen, Karin A. Mack, and Rita K. Noonan, "Slipping and Tripping: Fall Injuries in Adults Associated with Rugs and Carpets," *Journal of Injury and Violence Research* 5, no. 1 (January 2013): 61–69.

Chapter Five: People Matter Most

1. Vivek Murthy, "Work and the Loneliness Epidemic," *Harvard Business Review*, September 2017, https://hbr.org/cover-story/2017/09/work-and-the-loneliness-epidemic.

2. Yuval N. Harari, *Sapiens: A Brief History of Humankind* (New York: Harper, 2015), 21.

3. All data points in this paragraph taken from Michael Gerson, "Myths, Meaning, and Homo Sapiens," *Washington Post*, June 11, 2015, https://www.washingtonpost.com/opinions/myths-meaning-and-homo-sapiens/2015/06/11/28660902-106f-11e5-a0dc-2b6f404ff5cf_story.html?utm_term=.6b56a3e5ce0b.

4. Jared Diamond, *Collapse: How Societies Choose to Fail or Succeed* (New York: Viking, 2005).

5. See, for example, the following: Johann Hari, *Lost Connections: Uncovering the Real Causes of Depression—and the Unexpected Solutions* (New York: Bloomsbury, 2018); Susan Pinker, *The Village Effect: How Face-to-Face Contact Can Make Us Healthier and Happier* (Toronto: Vintage Canada, 2015).

6. See, for example, Dean Falk's "Prelinguistic Evolution in Early Hominins: Whence Motherese?" and the various responses to this piece contained in *Behavioral and Brain Sciences* 27 (2004): 491–541.

7. Sherry Turkle, *Reclaiming Conversation: The Power of Talk in a Digital Age* (New York: Penguin Press, 2015), 9.

8. Michaeleen Doucleff, "Are Hunter-Gatherers the Happiest Humans to Inhabit Earth?" NPR (October 1, 2017), https://www.npr.org/sections/goatsandsoda/2017/10/01/551018759/are-hunter-gatherers-the-happiest-humans-to-inhabit-earth; University of Cambridge, "Farmers Have Less Leisure Time Than Hunter-Gatherers," ScienceDaily (May 21, 2019), www.sciencedaily.com/releases/2019/05/190520115646.htm.

9. See, for example, Brandon H. Hidaka, "Depression as a Disease of Modernity: Explanations for Increasing Prevalence," *Journal of Affective Disorders* 140, no. 3 (November 2012): 205–14.

10. Steven Pinker, *The Better Angels of Our Nature: Why Violence Has Declined* (New York: Penguin, 2012).

11. For more on this general topic, see Antonia Ypsilanti et al.'s 2018 research: Susan Krauss Whitbourne, "5 Ways to Keep Loneliness From Turning into Depression," *Psychology Today*, November 10, 2018, https://www.psychologytoday.com/intl/blog/fulfillment-any-age/201811/5-ways-keep-loneliness-turning-depression.

12. For a more granular perspective on the rise of urbanization see Hannah Ritchie and Max Roser, "Urbanization," *Our World in Data* (September 2018), https://ourworldindata.org/urbanization.

13. R. I. M. Dunbar, "Neocortex Size as a Constraint on Group Size in Primates," *Journal of Human Evolution* 22, no. 6 (June 1992): 469–93, https://doi.org/10.1016/0047-2484(92)90081-J.

14. Aleks Krotoski, "Robin Dunbar: We Can Only Ever Have 150 Friends at Most . . ." *Guardian*, March 13, 2010, https://www.theguardian.com/technology/2010/mar/14/my-bright-idea-robin-dunbar.

15. Susan Tardanico, "Is Social Media Sabotaging Real Communication?" *Forbes*, April 30, 2012, https://www.forbes.com/sites/susantardanico/2012/04/30/is-social-media-sabotaging-real-communication/#21a6352b2b62.

16. Scott Barry Kaufman, "What Does It Mean to Be Self-Actualized in the 21st Century?" *Scientific American*, November 7, 2018, https://blogs.scientificamerican.com/beautiful-minds/what-does-it-mean-to-be-self-actualized-in-the-21st-century/; ———, "Who Created Maslow's Iconic Pyramid?" *Scientific American*, April 23, 2019, https://blogs.scientificamerican.com/beautiful-minds/who-created-maslows-iconic-pyramid/.

17. Barbara L. Fredrickson et al., "A Functional Genomic Perspective on Human Well-Being," *Proceedings of the National Academy of Sciences* (July 2013), doi: 10.1073/pnas.1305419110; Antonella Delle Fave et al., "The Eudaimonic and Hedonic Components of Happiness: Qualitative and Quantitative Findings," *Social Indicators Research* 100, no. 2 (January 2011): 185–207.

18. J. B. Grubbs and J. J. Exline, "Trait Entitlement: A Cognitive-Personality Source of Vulnerability to Psychological Distress," *Psychological Bulletin* 142, no. 11 (November 2016): 1204–26.

19. Toshimasa Sone et al., "Sense of Life Worth Living (Ikigai) and Mortality in Japan: Ohsaki Study," *Psychosomatic Medicine* 70, no. 6 (July 2008): 709, doi: 10.1097/PSY.0b013e31817e7e64.

20. Brené Brown, *The Gifts of Imperfection: Let Go of Who You Think You're Supposed to Be and Embrace Who You Are* (Center City, Minnesota: Hazelden Publishing, 2010), 6.

Chapter Six: Anchors

1. For this description and the following paraphrases and quotations I rely on Baya Voce, "The Simple Cure for Loneliness," YouTube video, TEDxSaltLakeCity, 13.27, posted October 7, 2016, https://www.youtube.com/watch?v=KSXh1YfNyVA.

2. R. Christ Fraley, "Adult Attachment Theory and Research," Department of Psychology University of Illinois at Urbana-Champaign, accessed September 17, 2019, http://labs.psychology.illinois.edu/~rcfraley/attachment.htm.

3. As Harry Harlow underscored in his classical work on material bonding and separation: "Harlow's Classic Studies Revealed the Importance of Maternal Contact," Association for Psychological Science, accessed September 17, 2019, https://www.psychologicalscience.org/publications/observer/obsonline/harlows-classic-studies-revealed-the-importance-of-maternal-contact.html. See also Sarah Gibbens, "Is Maternal Instinct Only for Moms? Here's the Science," *National Geographic*, May 9, 2018, https://www.nationalgeographic.com/news/2018/05/mothers-day-2018-maternal-instinct-oxytocin-babies-science/, for new research on the importance of oxytocin release among different types of caregivers.

4. Thomas Groennebaek and Kristian Vissing, "Impact of Resistance Training on Skeletal Muscle Mitochondrial Biogenesis, Content, and Function," *Frontiers in Physiology* (September 15, 2017 online publication), doi: 10.3389/fphys.2017.00713.

5. Perhaps no single figure did more to promote and celebrate the selfish theory as Ayn Rand: Eric Michael Johnson, "Ayn Rand vs. the Pygmies," *Slate*, October 3, 2012, https://slate.com/technology/2012/10/groups-and-gossip-drove-the-evolution-of-human-natur6. e.html.

Chapter Seven: Pivot to Heal: Fall and Therapeutic Winter

1. Denise Mann, "Alcohol and a Good Night's Sleep Don't Mix," WebMD (January 22, 2013), https://www.webmd.com/sleep-disorders/news/20130118/alcohol-sleep#1.

2. The following are a great place to start: Bessel A. van der Kolk, *The Body Keeps the Score: Brain, Mind, and Body in the Healing of Trauma* (New York: Penguin, 2015) and Gabor Maté, *In the Realm of Hungry Ghosts: Close Encounters With Addiction* (London: Vermilion, 2018).

Chapter Eight: Your Life Beyond

1. Linda Carroll, *Love Cycles: The Five Essential Stages of Lasting Love* (California: New World Library, 2014).

2. Esther Perel, *Mating in Captivity* (HarperCollins e-Books, 2014).

3. V. Volynets et al., "Intestinal Barrier Function and the Gut Microbiome Are Dif-

ferentially Affected in Mice Fed a Western-Style Diet or Drinking Water Supplemented with Fructose," *Journal of Nutrition* 147, no. 5 (May 2017), doi: 10.3945/jn.116.242859.

4. Keely A. Muscatell et al., "Exposure to an Inflammatory Challenge Enhances Neural Sensitivity to Negative and Positive Social Feedback," *Brain, Behavior, and Immunity* 57 (October 2016), doi: 10.1016/j.bbi.2016.03.022.

5. Philip Hunter, "The Inflammation Theory of Disease," *EMBO Reports* 13, no. 11 (November 2012): 968–70.

INDEX

Index

astronauts, 89

attachments, attachment theory, 133–34, 138, 147

attention economy, 137

autoimmune conditions, 208

autumn, *see* fall

B

Bastille Day terrorist attack, 133

BBC Research, 29

bears, 66–67

biomechanics, 84, 135

blood pressure, 8

Blue Zones, 68, 133

body rhythms, biological rhythms, 6, 7, 11
    circadian, *see* circadian rhythms
    endogenous, 6, 8
    in energy levels, 5
    exogenous, 7
    neuroscience of, 9–11
    ultradian, 8

body temperature, 6–7, 8, 28, 34

bones, 89, 91
    density of, 88, 89

Bowman, Katy, 84, 135

brain, 148
    amygdala in, 203
    hormones in, 10, 11
    light and, 32
    melatonin and, 10
    neurons in, 12, 15, 37
    and neuroscience of rhythms, 9–11
    neurotransmitters and, *see* neurotransmitters
    social group size and, 119

Brown, Brené, 123

Bushmen, 113

C

caffeine, 23, 24, 160, 182

calories, 57, 60, 63, 65, 91

cancer, 7, 36

carbohydrates, 15, 16, 17, 24, 44–48, 50, 52–54, 56–60, 66, 67, 130, 136, 164–65, 177, 188

cardiovascular disease (heart disease), 7, 46, 90, 95, 96, 208

cardiovascular fitness, 87, 90–91, 94, 144, 168, 188

carotenoids, 47

Carroll, Linda, 195

carrying and lifting movements, 77, 78, 87–88, 92, 94, 96–97, 131, 144

CDC, 25

change, resistance to, 182

Chasing the Sun: The Astonishing Science of Sunlight and How to Survive in a 24/7 World (Geddes), 31

children:
    movement and physical fitness in, 75–76
    parenting, 134, 174

Christmas, 200–201

circadian rhythms, xvi, xxvii, 8, 9, 16, 33, 40, 41, 139, 142, 144, 180
    eating and, 63–64, 66–67

cities, 107–8, 118
    urbanization, 106, 107, 114, 117

climate, 3
    rhythms in, 5

climate change, 60–61

clock, master, in humans and other mammals, 9, 34, 63, 65

clocks, 3, 140, 142, 161

CNN, 75

coffee shops, 118, 146

cognitive revolution, 104–5

collagen, 23, 208

Collapse (Diamond), 107

communication:
    biological cues in, 108–9

language, 104, 108
text messages, 102, 110, 120, 123
community(ies), 14, 102, 110, 115
in cities, 107–8
disconnection from, 118–21, 153
tribal groups, xi–xiv, 5, 78, 107, 113,
114, 119, 125
see also social connection
comparing ourselves to others, 37, 137
concrete, 87
connection, xvi, xix, xx, xxvii, 101–26,
120, 148, 158, 217
fall pivot and, 169–76
see also disconnection; social
connection
consumption and accumulation, 112–13,
173, 200–201, 210, 211
contraction and expansion, xiii–xiv, 5,
17–18
coregulation, 109
cortisol, 23, 24, 28, 36–37, 39, 152, 208
melatonin and, 36–37
cravings, xxviii, 16, 17, 39–41, 71,
164–65, 177
creativity, 8, 112
CrossFit, 85, 99, 145, 168
cycles, 3
cytokines, 89

D
darkness, 27–29, 40, 41, 131
light/dark cycle, 9, 33, 64,
139
melatonin and, 10, 28
see also light
death, 102, 179, 212–14
depression, 38, 40, 41, 102, 113–14,
125, 179, 188
dessert, 163–65
diabetes, 7, 53, 65
Diamond, Jared, 107

diet, *see* food
disconnection, 115–21, 188
from community, 118–21,
153
from nature, 107, 114, 117–18
from purpose, 121–22
from self, 116–17
see also connection
diseases and illnesses, xv, 10, 17, 113–14,
208
diurnal rhythm, 9–10, 33
DNA, xiii
dopamine, 11–12, 13, 16, 18, 24, 28,
39–40, 41, 80, 112, 136, 158
drug addiction, 18
Dunbar, Robin, 119–20
dynapenia, 89

E
Easter Island, 107
eating, *see* food
Egypt, 46
elders, elderly, 6
loneliness and, 99
movement and, 89,
98–99
risk of falls in, 98–99
electronics, 11, 140
emotions, 211
avoiding, 179
grief and sadness, 174–75, 176, 179,
213
healing of, 178
support for, 135
empathy, 109, 112
endorphins, 13, 152
endotoxin, 203
energy, 8, 40–41, 67
body temperature and, 6–7
rhythms in, 5
yearly fluctuations in, 6

Index

Index

ABOUT THE AUTHOR

Dallas Hartwig is the coauthor of the *New York Times* bestsellers *The Whole30* and *It Starts with Food*. A functional medicine practitioner and physical therapist, he's also the cohost of *The Living Experiment* podcast and the author of a popular email newsletter on healthy living. He has been featured in media such as the *Today* show, *Good Morning America*, *The Dr. Oz Show*, *The View*, and more. He lives in Salt Lake City. To learn more, visit dallashartwig.com and @dallashartwig on Instagram.